jan 616 825
EME

2015

Table of Contents

Practice Test #1

Practice Questions

1. Which of the following is NOT a sign of labored breathing?
    a. Diminished breath sounds
    b. Use of accessory muscles to breathe
    c. An adult with a respiratory rate of 12 breaths per minute
    d. An infant with a respiratory rate of 12 breaths per minute

2. You come across a scene where the patient appears to be in respiratory distress and is making a gurgling noise. You immediately know that you need to
    a. Intubate the patient
    b. Suction the patient immediately
    c. Log-roll the patient
    d. Perform chest thrusts on the patient

3. Which of the following would be the most appropriate choice for positioning an unresponsive patient with suspected trauma?
    a. Jaw thrust technique
    b. Head-tilt chin-lift technique
    c. Triple-airway maneuver
    d. Side-facing chin-lift technique

4. Which of the following is NOT a true statement?
    a. The oropharyngeal airway should be selected for an unconscious patient
    b. The oropharyngeal airway is a better choice for a patient who is having seizures
    c. A conscious patient is likely to experience the gag reflex with the use of an oropharyngeal airway
    d. The nasopharyngeal airway is less likely to stimulate the gag reflex

5. What is the preferred method of ventilation in the field for a patient who is not able to breathe on his own?
    a. Mouth-to-mouth ventilation
    b. Mouth-to-mask ventilation
    c. Two-person bag-valve-mask
    d. One-person bag-valve-mask

6. Which of the following would be considered an indicator of adequate ventilation?
    a. The patient's skin has a bluish tinge
    b. The patient has a heart rate of 120 beats per minute
    c. The patient has a distended abdomen
    d. The patient is being ventilated a minimum of 12 times per minute

7. Which of the following would be most important when attempting to ventilate a patient with facial trauma?
    a. Tilt the head back to properly ventilate the patient
    b. Establish a nasal airway immediately
    c. Have a suctioning device close by in case significant blood or vomit needs to be suctioned out of the airway
    d. Consider a tracheotomy in the field if facial trauma is excessive and bleeding and swelling are present

8. Which of the following statements best describes what should be done with dentures during airway management?
    a. The dentures should be left in place if possible to help the mouth retain form
    b. The dentures should be removed immediately to prevent airway obstruction
    c. Remove the dentures if the patient is unconscious
    d. It doesn't really matter

9. Which of the following set of baseline vital signs would be most concerning to you?
    a. A 12-year-old boy with a pulse of 110, respiratory rate of 20, and blood pressure of 95/60
    b. A newborn baby with a pulse of 155, respiratory rate of 52, and blood pressure of 85/40
    c. A 3-year-old girl with a pulse of 80, respiratory rate of 30, and blood pressure of 82/45
    d. A 16-year-old boy with a pulse of 100, respiratory rate of 25, and blood pressure of 100/60

10. Which of the following terms refers to a high-pitched sound made during inspiration?
    a. Grunting
    b. Stridor
    c. Wheezing
    d. Crowing

11. The medical terminology for breathing too fast and shallow is
    a. Bradypnea
    b. Dyspnea
    c. Tachypnea
    d. Bronchiectasis

12. You arrive on the scene following a call for respiratory distress. The patient appears to be thin, barrel-chested, and breathing through pursed lips. You notice an oxygen tank nearby. Your immediate assessment is
    a. Emphysema
    b. Chronic bronchitis
    c. Asthma
    d. Pneumonia

13. The patient requests assistance with administering her asthma medication. Which of the following would not be an appropriate step to take?
    a. Obtain authorization from the physician before administering the dose
    b. Check with the patient to determine when the last dose was taken
    c. Check the temperature of the inhaler because a cold inhaler may not provide the appropriate dose
    d. Administer the dose immediately, as the patient's respiratory status appears to be worsening

14. Types of bronchodilators include all of the following EXCEPT:
   a. Alupent
   b. Pulmicort
   c. Proventil
   d. Metaprel

15. Which of the following is the most important statement about treating patients with respiratory distress?
   a. Oxygen should be administered immediately
   b. A spacer should always be used with inhalers
   c. Medical authorization should be obtained before administering an inhaler
   d. Immediately begin the focused history and physical in order to determine what you are dealing with

16. An important anatomical landmark when performing the Sellick maneuver is the
   a. Trachea
   b Esophagus
   c. Cricoid ring
   d. Diaphragmatic ring

17. All of the following are indications for using endotracheal intubation EXCEPT:
   a. A patient experiencing a medical crisis, such as a cardiac arrest that is unable to protect their airway
   b. A patient who is unresponsive except to painful stimuli
   c. A patient with apnea with whom you are having difficulty establishing an airway
   d. A patient with an absent gag reflex

18. As you prepare to place an endotracheal tube, all of the following are important steps to take before placing the endotracheal tube EXCEPT:
   a. Put on gloves, mask, and eye protection protect yourself from potentially hazardous bodily fluids
   b. Check the cuff for possible leaks by inflating the balloon and squeezing gently to make sure air is not escaping
   c. Insert the stylus into the tube
   d. Select the proper tube diameter, which in most cases is an 8.5 to 9 mm diameter

19. What is the name of the tool that is used to help visualize the airway during intubation?
   a. Endoscope
   b. Laryngoscope
   c. Bronchoscope
   d. Thorascope

20. After you have used the laryngoscope to intubate the patient, you need to check placement of the endotracheal tube. Breath sounds are not audible in the area of the lungs, but you do hear a gurgling sound. How do you interpret this type of noise?
    a. The endotracheal tube is in the proper position
    b. The endotracheal tube is almost in the correct position, but it needs to be advanced a few millimeters more
    c. The endotracheal tube is located in the esophagus
    d. The endotracheal tube needs to be pulled back by a few millimeters

21. You have successfully paced an endotracheal tube into the patient. You have confirmed placement with different techniques. The patient is now stable and ready to be transported to the hospital. The patient is loaded onto the ambulance. As you begin to head to the hospital, the patient's oxygen saturation level begins to drop as well as the heart rate. What should you immediately suspect is the issue?
    a. The patient is going into cardiac arrest
    b. The endotracheal tube has dislodged and is no longer in the proper position
    c. The patient possibly has pneumonia
    d. The patient needs to quickly reach the emergency room so additional medical care can be provided

22. Which of the following is a correct statement about circulation?
    a. Oxygen-poor blood flows into the left atrium, then the left ventricle through the pulmonary arteries to the lungs to receive oxygen, then into the pulmonary veins to the right atrium into the right ventricle, and then it is pumped to the rest of the body
    b. Oxygen-poor blood flows into the right ventricle, then the right atrium through the pulmonary arteries to the lungs to receive oxygen, then into the pulmonary veins to the left ventricle into the left atrium, and then it is pumped to the rest of the body
    c. Oxygen-poor blood flows into the right atrium, then the right ventricle through the pulmonary arteries to the lungs to receive oxygen, then into the pulmonary veins to the left atrium into the left ventricle, and then it is pumped to the rest of the body
    d. Oxygen-poor blood flows into the right atrium, then the right ventricle through the pulmonary veins to the lungs to receive oxygen, then into the pulmonary arteries to the left ventricle into the left atrium, and then it is pumped to the rest of the body

23. What is the name of the major artery located in the neck?
    a. Carotid
    b. Aorta
    c. Femoral
    d. Superior vena cava

24. You receive a request to respond to a call from a 52-year-old woman who is complaining of chest pain and trouble breathing. When you arrive on the scene, what is the first step you should take?
    a. Give the patient a dose of nitroglycerin
    b. Assess the severity of the patient's pain
    c. Administer high-flow oxygen
    d. Obtain the patient's blood pressure

25. Which of the following would NOT be a contraindication for administering nitroglycerin to a male patient having chest pain?
    a. The patient does not have a prescription for nitroglycerin
    b. The patient's wife tells you her husband used Cialis the night before.
    c. The patient's blood pressure is 110/75 mmHg
    d. The patient has his own prescription for nitroglycerin, but you have not received authorization from the physician to administer it

26. Which of the following is likely to be the sublingual dosage for nitroglycerin?
    a. 0.3 mg
    b. 0.1 mg
    c. 3 mg
    d. 1 g

27. The American Heart Association defines the sequence of links in the chain of survival as:
    a. Early CPR, early recognition and access to EMS, early defibrillation, and early access to ACLS
    b. Early recognition and access to EMS, early CPR, early defibrillation, and early access to ACLS
    c. Early defibrillation, early access to ACLS, early CPR, early recognition, and access to EMS
    d. Early recognition and access to EMS, early defibrillation, early CPR, and early access to ACLS

28. In which of the following conditions would the use of an AED be most effective?
    a. Atrial fibrillation
    b. Asystole
    c. Ventricular tachycardia with a pulse
    d. Ventricular fibrillation

29. Which of the following steps is NOT considered standard operating procedure for using an AED?
    a. For an unwitnessed cardiac arrest, perform five cycles of CPR, and then apply the AED
    b. For a witnessed cardiac arrest in an adult, apply the AED immediately
    c. Continue to apply shocks until the pulse is regained, but alternate with cycles of CPR
    d. Apply two shocks, and then wait for the AED to provide a message on how to proceed

30. Once you have shocked a patient who is in cardiac arrest, what should be done next?
    a. Restart CPR
    b. Check for the presence of a pulse
    c. Call the physician for direction
    d. Start chest compressions

31. What should be done if a patient goes into cardiac arrest while being transported to the hospital?
    a. The driver should stop the ambulance immediately in order to use the AED appropriately
    b. Attach the AED and deliver a shock if directed to
    c. Initiate CPR and wait until you arrive at the hospital where ALS can be initiated
    d. Administer high-flow oxygen and begin chest compressions

32. Which of the following would NOT be considered characteristic of someone who is in shock?
    a. Rapid pulse
    b. Hypoperfusion
    c. High blood pressure
    d. Paleness

33. When you are assessing a patient who has been in a car accident without signs of obvious trauma or bleeding, which of the following signs would be MOST concerning to you?
    a. Respiratory rate of 15 breaths per minute
    b. Pulse rate of 100
    c. Blood pressure of 115/78
    d. The patient begins to move around the stretcher and tries to get up, asking when she can leave

34. What is the potential effect of beta-blockers on the symptoms of shock?
    a. Causes blood pressure to drop
    b. Lowers blood pressure and keeps the heart rate steady
    c. Lowers blood pressure and lowers heart rate
    d. No effect

35. In providing emergency care for a patient with shock, after putting on appropriate bodily substance precautions, what are most important steps to follow next?
    a. Stop the bleeding and prevent heat loss
    b. Assess the airway/ventilate and stop the bleeding
    c. Assess the airway/ventilate and prevent heat loss
    d. Stop the bleeding and transport immediately

36. Why is it important for a patient in shock to remain warm?
    a. To prevent oxygen from being wasted as shivering occurs
    b. The patient will respond better to treatment if warm
    c. To help maintain blood pressure
    d. To keep the patient comfortable

37. A patient you are treating presents with a wound on his leg. You notice the blood is bright red and is spurting out from the wound. What kind of bleed is this most likely to be?
    a. Deep muscle bleed
    b. Capillary bleed
    c. Venous bleed
    d. Arterial bleed

38. What would be the appropriate pressure point in order to reduce bleeding in the patient with a leg wound?
    a. Temporal artery
    b. Carotid artery
    c. Femoral artery
    d. Brachial artery

39. Which of the following statements is NOT true regarding the use of a tourniquet?
    a. The tourniquet is considered to be a last-resort way to treat bleeding
    b. A tourniquet should be placed directly over a joint to maximize its effectiveness
    c. Once a tourniquet is applied, it should not be taken off, because it may cause blood clots to mobilize
    d. The tourniquet should be plainly visible, so anyone else who comes to treat the patient will easily see it

40. You have been called to the home of a patient who was found unconscious. On first observation, you notice the patient has vomited what appears to be vomit mixed with dark brown liquid that looks like coffee grounds. This could possibly be indicative of which of the following?
    a. Blood that was swallowed from a wound in the mouth
    b. Bleeding that is originating from an internal bleed in the stomach
    c. Blood that has been in the stomach for a while and has been partially digested
    d. Blood that is originating from a lower gastrointestinal bleed

41. If you suspect a patient is bleeding internally, which of the following would NOT be the best course of action to take?
    a. Apply a pneumatic antishock garment and inflate to prevent further abdominal bleeding
    b. Transport immediately
    c. Apply direct pressure to an injury on the extremity to slow the bleeding, and then splint the injury
    d. Ensure a patent airway and administer high-flow oxygen

42. An 82-year-old female patient is complaining of abdominal pain, difficulty breathing, feeling extremely tired, and dizziness. These symptoms may be indicative of
    a. Abdominal bleeding
    b. Influenza
    c. Asthma
    d. Myocardial infarction

43. You are assessing a pregnant patient who appears to be close to term. She is having regular contractions, and upon examination, you decide she is in the second stage of labor. What would be the BEST indication of this?
    a. Regular contractions 10 minutes apart
    b. Evidence of bloody show
    c. Crowning is evident
    d. The cervix is dilated almost to 10 cm

44. The woman in the previous case tells you she needs to go to the bathroom immediately to move her bowels. What should you do?
    a. Walk her to the nearest bathroom, but stand outside the door in case she needs assistance
    b. Do not allow her to go to the bathroom
    c. Wait until the next contraction is finished, and then allow her to go to the bathroom
    d. Ask her to wait a few minutes then reassess

45. A woman in her 34th week of pregnancy presents with vaginal bleeding. From your EMT training, you know this type of bleeding is likely indicative of
    a. An issue with the placenta
    b. Premature delivery
    c. Impending miscarriage
    d. Preeclampsia

46. How long is the average length of a woman's first labor?
    a. 10 to 12 hours
    b. 12 to 18 hours
    c. 18 to 20 hours
    d. 18 to 24 hours

47. The baby's head is crowning, and you begin to prepare for imminent delivery. Which of the following would NOT be an appropriate action during delivery?
    a. Set up a sterile field using sterile towels or paper barriers
    b. Loosen the umbilical cord if it is wrapped around the baby's neck
    c. Carefully break the amniotic sac if it is still intact
    d. Press gently on the fontanelles in order to prevent tearing of the perineum

48. What position is the head of the baby in most deliveries?
    a. The head can be in any direction
    b. Head facing sideways
    c. Head facing down
    d. Head facing up

49. All of the following are true statements about the third stage of labor EXCEPT:
    a. The placenta should be discarded after delivery
    b. The placenta will be delivered within 30 minutes
    c. The woman can be transported to the hospital before the placenta is delivered
    d. Pieces of the placenta can remain attached to the uterine wall and may cause bleeding

50. An infant born with your assistance should have APGAR scores assessed at which of the following intervals?
    a. Immediately following birth and at 5 minutes
    b. 1 minute of life and at 5 minutes
    c. 2 minutes of life and at 8 minutes
    d. 5 minutes of life and at 10 minutes

51. As you are assessing an infant's APGAR scores, you realize that the infant's heart rate is 78 beats per minute. What should you do next?
   a. Provide artificial ventilations at a rate of 15 liters per minute then reassess after 30 seconds
   b. Provide positive pressure ventilations at a rate of 30 to 60 per minute then reassess after 30 seconds
   c. Start chest compressions according to newborn standards, and reassess in 1 minute. If the heart rate is above 100 beats per minute, stop the compressions and administer high-flow oxygen via a nonrebreather mask
   d. Start chest compressions according to newborn standards, and reassess after 30 seconds. If the heart rate is above 100 beats per minute, stop the compressions and administer free-flow oxygen

52. All of the following are appropriate steps to take in delivering a baby with a prolapsed cord EXCEPT:
   a. Gently try to push the umbilical cord back into the birth canal
   b. Position the mother so her head is facing down, and slightly elevate the pelvis
   c. Try to push the baby off the umbilical cord using several fingers of a gloved hand gently inserted into the vagina
   d. Apply damp and sterile dressings to the portion of the umbilical cord that can be seen outside the birth canal

53. You are assisting with the delivery of an infant thought to have a gestational age of approximately 33 weeks. Which of the following would be true for all premature infants?
   a. Premature infants will need to be intubated upon delivery to assist with delivery
   b. Premature delivery that occurs outside of a hospital will likely end in the death of the baby
   c. Premature infants are likely to have a drop in their body temperature quickly due to the lack of body fat
   d. Judgment should be used as to whether to resuscitate a baby based on appearance and size

54. You are attempting to oxygenate a four-year-old child who is resisting having the oxygen mask placed on his face. What would an alternate be to oxygenate this child?
   a. Nonrebreather mask
   b. Ambu Bag
   c. Nasal prongs
   d. Blow-by

55. Which of the following is an example of what you would NOT do if you suspect a three-year-old child has a foreign body airway obstruction?
   a. Visualize the airway, and remove the foreign object using a finger sweep if you are able
   b. Perform back blows
   c. Perform abdominal thrusts
   d. If the child is not breathing and is unresponsive, give two breaths, then look for a foreign body in the airway

56. You are responding to a 911 call for a child having a seizure. After making sure the child's airway is patent, what is the most appropriate course of action?
   a. Make sure the child does not hurt himself during the seizure. After the seizure is done, position the child in the recovery position and administer oxygen
   b. Call for ALS backup
   c. Position the child in the recovery position, and then administer antiseizure medication. Wait for the seizure to subside
   d. Make sure the child does not hurt himself during the seizure. Insert a mouth guard into the child's mouth to protect him or her from injury. Administer oxygen

57. You are responding to a call for a near-drowning. You arrive at the lake and discover a 12-year-old boy is being pulled to shore by a couple of bystanders. What should you do to help?
   a. Immediately jump into the water to provide assistance in removing the boy from the water
   b. Wait until the bystanders get closer, and then help pull the boy from the water
   c. Immobilize the boy before removing him from the water in case of possible spinal damage
   d. Allow the bystanders to pull the boy out of the water, immobilize him, and then move to a dry area so you can assess him

58. You are providing treatment to an eight-year-old girl who dropped a burning marshmallow on her leg while near a campfire. The injury appears to be approximately two inches in diameter and no more severe than a second-degree burn. What is the proper treatment for a burn injury?
   a. Cover the burn injury with dry sterile gauze dressings
   b. Cover the burn injury with sterile dressings that have been dampened
   c. Cover the injury with butter or other available ointment
   d. Apply ice directly to the burn

59. You are evaluating a three-month-old infant. The father reports the baby had been very irritable and inconsolable earlier in the day but now has been lethargic. There are no obvious signs of injury. The infant's respiratory rate is 22 breaths per minute. The infant has not woken up to eat. What condition may be a possibility?
   a. Seizure disorder
   b. Shaken baby syndrome
   c. Pneumonia
   d. Cardiac defect

60. When confronted with a possible case of child abuse, such as shaken baby syndrome, which of the following is the most appropriate course of action?
   a. Tell the parents you suspect child abuse or shaken baby syndrome
   b. Immediately call the police, and wait for a response
   c. Begin to administer medical care, and transport the child after police arrive
   d. Administer appropriate medical care, transport the child immediately, and communicate objective information to the hospital

61. A child with developmental delays has a tracheostomy tube inserted to help him breathe at home. The tracheostomy tube has become dislodged, and the parents have not been able to replace it. The child is going into respiratory distress. What should you do before the patient is transported?
   a. Try to put the tracheostomy tube back in yourself
   b. Perform CPR
   c. Cover the stoma and ventilate with a bag-valve-mask over the mouth and nose
   d. Ventilate through the stoma with a bag-valve-mask

62. You arrive on the scene to treat a child who is having difficulty breathing. The mother is crying and appears hysterical. What is the best course of action?
   a. Try to reassure the mother, ask her to breathe deeply to calm down, and explain that the child will respond better to treatment if the parents are calm
   b. Ask the mother to leave the room until she calms down
   c. Offer a sedative to help her calm down
   d. Tell the mother sternly to stop crying

63. All of the following are symptoms of hypoglycemia EXCEPT:
   a. Hunger
   b. Sweating
   c. Frequent urination
   d. Confusion or disorientation

64. In a patient with known diabetes experiencing hypoglycemia, what is the appropriate initial treatment if the patient is alert?
   a. Have the patient drink 16 ounces of orange juice
   b. Administer one full tube of oral glucose
   c. Administer glucagon
   d. Administer epinephrine

65. All of the following are medications used to treat diabetes EXCEPT:
   a. Atenolol
   b. Insulin
   c. Glucotrol
   d. Starlix

66. Common symptoms of an allergic reaction may include all of the following EXCEPT:
   a. Nausea, vomiting or diarrhea
   b. Swelling of the tongue, face, or hands
   c. Difficulty breathing or swallowing
   d. Hypertension and pruritus

67. What is the name of the medication given to help reverse a severe allergic reaction?
   a. Norepinephrine
   b. Epinephrine
   c. Fexofenadine
   d. Fluticasone

68. You are evaluating a patient who was found unconscious. You notice an odor of petroleum on the patient's breath. What could this odor indicate to you?
   a. The patient has consumed a petroleum-based product
   b. The patient is having a diabetic emergency
   c. It likely does not mean anything
   d. The patient has ingested pesticide

69. All of the following are considerations for possible inhaled toxins EXCEPT:
   a. Inhaled toxins can cause difficulty breathing and airway swelling
   b. Inhaled toxins are not as quickly absorbed; therefore, the consequences are not as great as with ingested toxins
   c. Inhaled toxins can be present in the air and may affect others in the immediate area
   d. Inhaled toxins can cause fainting or seizures

70. Activated charcoal works by:
   a. Inducing vomiting
   b. Intravenously binds the toxin, as it is absorbed to prevent side effects
   c. Binding the toxin in the gut to prevent absorption
   d. Works to bind acid- or alkali-type toxic substances in the gut

71. You are providing emergency care to a hypothermic patient. All of the following are appropriate treatment steps EXCEPT:
   a. Allow the patient to walk to a warmer place
   b. Cover the patient with as many blankets as are available
   c. Utilize heat packs wrapped in towels around the armpits, neck, head, and groin areas
   d. Provide warm, humidified oxygen

72. You are treating a patient with a cold injury to the right hand. Transport to the nearest hospital will take 20 to 30 minutes. What is the most effective method of treating this patient?
   a. Apply heat packs to the affected hand
   b. Put the patient's hand in water that has been warmed to 102 to 104 °F during the ambulance ride
   c. Gently massage the hand during transport
   d. Apply warm, wet dressings over the hand

73. Which of the following correctly describes a condition where the patient's internal body temperature is greater than 98.6 °F?
   a. Heat stroke
   b. Heat exhaustion
   c. Hyperaridity
   d. Hyperthermia

74. You are responding to a 911 call for an elderly woman who has fallen. When you enter the home, a family member who cares for the patient leads you to her bedroom. As you begin to examine the patient, you notice old bruises all over her body, and it looks as though she has had black eyes recently. You notice she seems reluctant to talk to you and continues to glance over at the family member present in the room. As part of your evaluation, you note:
    a. The patient appears to be clumsy
    b. Possible prescription medication abuse
    c. Possible need for long-term care placement
    d. Possible elder abuse

75. You are responding to a 911 call for a 40-year-old man who may possibly be having a psychotic episode. When you enter the scene, which of the following would you LEAST likely do first?
    a. Position yourself in the room so you are close to an exit and the patient is not in the middle, blocking your path
    b. Scan the room for objects that could potentially be used as weapons
    c. Ask the patient about his medical history
    d. Obtain information from family or people present who can give background information

76. After evaluating and trying to calm an agitated patient, you decide that restraints are necessary. Which of the following is NOT a correct step in the restraint process?
    a. Position the patient stomach-down on the stretcher
    b. Before putting the restraints on, document the patient's condition, then continue to document the condition every few minutes
    c. Apply a surgical mask to the patient's mouth if the patient is attempting to bite you
    d. Assess the tightness of the restraints, and adjust as necessary for comfort

77. A 22-year-old man was riding his bicycle. He hit a bump and fell off his bike into the street. A passing car ran over his leg. What kind of leg injury did he likely sustain from the car?
    a. Laceration
    b. Contusion
    c. Avulsion
    d. Closed crush injury

78. All of the following are layers of the skin EXCEPT:
    a. Epidermis
    b. Sebaceous
    c. Dermis
    d. Subcutaneous

79. The appropriate care for a patient with a skewer stuck in his leg would be to:
    a. Control the bleeding, and bandage around the object to stabilize and secure in place
    b. Remove the object, and then control the bleeding with sterile dressings
    c. Try to get a feel for the object. If it is loose, pull it out, and then control the bleeding
    d. Irrigate the area, and then bandage with sterile dressings

80. If a patient has a tooth knocked completely out of her mouth, you should do all of the following EXCEPT:
   a. Make sure no other signs of injury are present
   b. Rinse the tooth off, and then place it in milk or normal saline
   c. Rinse the tooth off, and then place it inside the patient's mouth between the cheek and gumline if she is cooperative
   d. Hold the tooth by its root, rinse it off, and then place it in water

81. Which of the following is NOT an appropriate step in the emergency care of an adult burn patient with a moderate-size burn?
   a. Use cool, sterile wet dressings to cover the burned area
   b. Keep the patient warm
   c. Remove all jewelry as well as any clothing that may still be smoldering
   d. Use a sterile, dry dressing to cover the burned area

82. What is the very first step in treating a patient with an electrical burn?
   a. Run cool water over the burn to cool
   b. Apply Silvadene
   c. Make sure the source of the electrical burn has been disconnected
   d. Cover the area with a dry sterile dressing

83. The main bones in the leg are:
   a. Humerus, ulna, radius
   b. Carpals, metacarpals, phalanges
   c. Femur, fibula, tibia
   d. Clavicle, scapula, sternum

84. The name of the disease that causes thinning of the bones and loss of bone density is called
   a. Osteogenesis imperfecta
   b. Osteoporosis
   c. Paget's disease
   d. Osteosarcoma

85. A 26-year-old man has fractured his left tibia while playing softball. He is in extreme pain. You arrive on the scene. You have assessed his vital signs, and you immobilized the joints above and below the injury. There are no open wounds. What is the next step in treatment?
   a. Splint the radius the way you found it
   b. Gently try to realign the radius, and then apply the splint
   c. Apply ice packs to the area
   d. Transport the patient immediately

86. All of the following are immobilization devices used for spine or neck injuries EXCEPT:
   a. Cervical collar
   b. Long spine board
   c. Short backboard
   d. Thoracolumbar orthosis

87. When assessing a patient with a possible spinal injury, which of the following is something you should NEVER do?
    a. Ask the patient if he feels any areas of tenderness
    b. If the patient is not in pain, ask him to move his back to see what the response is
    c. Position yourself in front of the patient while asking him questions
    d. Ask the patient to grab your hands and squeeze

88. A diving injury is likely to cause which of the following injuries?
    a. Distraction injury
    b. Whiplash
    c. Compression injury
    d. Lateral bending injury

89. In a situation in which you need to use a long backboard or spinal board, how do you get the patient safely onto the board if she is lying down?
    a. Log-roll
    b. Gently slide the board under her
    c. Have a minimum of three EMTs lift the patient onto the board
    d. Standing take-down

90. The first step in immobilizing a patient using a Kendrick Extrication Device (KED) is
    a. Position the KED behind the patient's back, ensuring that it is centered with his spine
    b. Establish cervical stabilization using a cervical collar
    c. Assess and document distal pulses
    d. Lift the patient while he is still sitting, and place him on the long backboard

91. The proper order for securing the straps on the KED is
    a. Head, top, middle, bottom, legs
    b. Head, legs, top, middle, bottom
    c. Legs, head, top, bottom, middle
    d. Middle, bottom, legs, head, top

92. Signs of blood or fluid leakage from the nose or ears may be symptoms of
    a. Traumatic head injury
    b. Spinal cord injury
    c. Influenza
    d. Subarachnoid hemorrhage

93. A patient is involved in an accident, and she is wearing a helmet. All of the following are indications for removing the helmet to treat the patient EXCEPT:
    a. You are not able to monitor the patient's breathing adequately
    b. The patient requires spinal stabilization
    c. The helmet is loose and allows for the head to freely move
    d. The helmet is tight and does not allow the head to move freely

94. You are responding to a 911 call at the scene of a car accident. There appears to be two people in the car, and they are not able to get out. Which of the following is NOT an indication for rapid extrication?
    a. You smell gasoline around the car
    b. One of patient appears to be in severe pain
    c. The patient closest to you needs to be moved quickly in order to reach the second patient, who appears to be critically injured
    d. The patient appears to be in cardiac arrest

95. The acronym to use when performing a trauma assessment is
    a. DCAP-LETS
    b. CAP-BLT
    c. DCAP-BTLS
    d. BDIP-BTLS

96. The significance of distended jugular veins is
    a. Increase in pressure in the circulatory system
    b. Extreme loss of blood
    c. Dehydration
    d. Improper positioning of the patient

97. All of the following are basic supplies that all ambulances should be equipped with EXCEPT:
    a. Ballistic vests
    b. Suction equipment
    c. Splinting supplies
    d. AED

98. When responding to an emergency call in an ambulance with red lights and sirens activated, which of the following is NOT an acceptable procedure?
    a. Pay attention to weather and road conditions, as an ambulance can easily roll over
    b. All EMS personnel in the ambulance should wear a seat belt
    c. Always drive with the ambulance's headlights on
    d. Pass a school bus with its red lights flashing

99. Intermediate-level disinfection kills all of the following EXCEPT:
    a. Tuberculosis bacteria
    b. Bacterial spores
    c. Most viruses
    d. Most fungi

100. The minimum size requirement for a landing zone for helicopter transport is
    a. 100 feet by 100 feet
    b. 75 feet by 75 feet
    c. 60 feet by 60 feet
    d. 30 feet by 30 feet

101. All of the following would be acceptable situations where air transport would be indicated EXCEPT:
    a. 22-year-old male who fell off a balcony with probably head injury
    b. 62-year-old female with 50% burns on her lower extremities
    c. 30-year-old female in labor who is 50 miles from her designated delivery hospital when she presents in labor
    d. 55-year-old male involved in a motor vehicle accident and ejected from the vehicle

102. As an EMT, which of the following is NOT a typical step when dealing with a potential fire situation?
    a. Grab a fire extinguisher, and try to put out the fire
    b. Turn off the car ignition if the car is still running
    c. Ask bystanders to refrain from smoking
    d. Survey the scene to check for downed wires or fluid leakage from the car

103. Which of the following is not a TRUE statement regarding dealing with a potentially hazardous scene?
    a. When entering the scene, the wind direction should be determined, and the scene should be entered upwind
    b. If there is no apparent odor, the scene is likely safe
    c. The area should be cordoned off to isolate it from bystanders
    d. A copy of the book Emergency Response Guidebook should be on hand in the ambulance for quick reference

104. One public service agency resource that should be contacted early in the response to a hazardous chemical situation is:
    a. OSHA
    b. NFPA
    c. FDA
    d. CHEMTREC

105. The lowest priority injury in a triage situation would be:
    a. Severe burns with respiratory arrest
    b. Traumatic amputation
    c. Shock
    d. Cardiopulmonary arrest

106. The legal responsibility of a paid EMT to provide emergency medical care to a patient when requested is called:
    a. Duty to act
    b. Standards of care
    c. Good Samaritan law
    d. Code of ethics

107. In order for an EMT to be considered negligent, four criteria must be met. Which of the following is not considered one of the criteria?
    a. The EMT failed to provide emergency services
    b. The injury to the patient was directly caused by the omission of a specific treatment that would have helped the patient
    c. A delay in emergency treatment occurred due to inability to get through a traffic backup
    d. The EMT failed to provide the appropriate level of service that another EMT with similar education, training, and experience would have provided in the same type of case

108. Which of the following would be considered abandonment?
    a. You arrive at the emergency room and transfer care to the emergency room physician
    b. You ask the first responder to take over care of a patient for you who does not appear to be critically injured
    c. You are not able to safely enter a scene because of the odor of a noxious fume that you are not able to identify
    d. You arrive at the scene of a 911 call, but the patient's symptoms subside after a few minutes, and she declines treatment, so you leave

109. Which of the following individuals is least likely to give expressed consent?
    a. A 30-year-old who is legal guardian for a 10-year-old child
    b. A 45-year-old man with a blood alcohol level of over twice the legal limit
    c. A young woman who recently celebrated her 18th birthday
    d. A 75-year-old man with cancer and a do-not-resuscitate order

110. You have arrived onto the scene to respond to a 911 call for a child in respiratory distress. When you arrive, you discover that the parents are divorced, are arguing about providing care, and the father is blocking your access. What is the best course of action for you to take?
    a. Treat the child in the way that you see fit
    b. Physically remove the child from the situation, and try to treat in another area away from the parents
    c. Try to reason with the parents and explain the urgency of the situation
    d. Call the police for assistance

111. What is a possible outcome if an adult patient refuses treatment, but the EMT overrides this decision and transports the patient to the hospital anyway?
    a. The EMT could potentially face an assault and battery or kidnapping charge
    b. The patient may change their mind en route to the hospital
    c. The hospital will ultimately decide if the patient requires treatment
    d. The patient may survive the injury because of the EMT's actions and decision

112. If a mentally competent patient refuses treatment, even though he clearly requires treatment, what is the next best step?
    a. Accept the patient's refusal, and leave the scene
    b. Ask the emergency room doctor to come to the scene
    c. Carefully document the situation, and ask the patient to sign a release from liability form
    d. Ask a witness to sign a form to support you, in case the patient later sues

113. All of the following are considered advanced directives EXCEPT:
    a. Living will
    b. Durable power of attorney
    c. DNR order
    d. Expressed consent

114. You arrive on the scene to find an 80-year-old man in full cardiac arrest. The man's daughter tells you that he has a DNR order, but she is unable to provide verification of this. What should you do?
    a. Provide comfort care, and transport the patient to the hospital to verify the DNR order
    b. Begin CPR, because written documentation is required for a DNR order
    c. Attempt to contact the patient's primary care physician
    d. Try to contact other family members to verify the DNR order

115. Which of the following would be a violation of confidentiality?
    a. Providing information to a police officer for a suspected rape situation
    b. Giving a medical update to a neighbor who is on the scene while treatment is occurring
    c. Calling authorities to report that a patient has been bitten by a potentially rabid raccoon
    d. Providing information to the nurse admitting the patient in the emergency room

116. Which of the following statements is NOT true about HIPAA as it relates to EMS?
    a. HIPAA does not apply to healthcare providers who do not charge for their services
    b. HIPAA may be applicable to EMS systems if electronic bills are submitted for medical services provided
    c. HIPAA is directly applicable to EMS systems, because medical care is being provided
    d. The way HIPAA is applied to individual EMS systems is directed by the policies and procedures of each system

117. A patient is in full respiratory arrest and will likely not survive the arrest. The EMT learns the patient is an organ donor. What is the appropriate way to proceed?
    a. Continue to provide treatment at an appropriate level based on the patient's condition
    b. Immediately stop care, and provide comfort to the patient
    c. Contact the patient's family to pay their last respects
    d. Contact the medical director for advice on how to proceed

118. The purpose of a Medic Alert tag is:
    a. To convey a DNR order
    b. To direct the EMT to the patient's advanced directives
    c. To provide important information to EMT about the patient's medical condition
    d. To provide emergency contact information

119. Which of the following is NOT a recommended action when responding to an emergency call that is also a possible crime scene?
    a. Wait for the police to arrive
    b. Be careful when entering the scene, so potential evidence is not disturbed
    c. Document the reason for any delay in treatment
    d. Enter the scene immediately to begin emergency medical treatment for the patient

120. What is the appropriate agency to report to in case of an incident in which an EMT is stuck by a needle?
    a. OSHA
    b. FDA
    c. CDC
    d. NLRB

Answers and Explanations

1. C: A normal respiratory rate for an adult is between 12 to 20 breaths per minute. For children, the normal rate is 15 to 30 breaths per minute. An infant has a much higher respiratory rate, at 25 to 50 breaths per minute because the oxygen requirement for infants is much higher than that for an adult. Normal breathing results in both lungs inflating at the same rate. Breath sounds should be detected with the use of a stethoscope. If breath sounds are absent or diminished, breathing difficulties should immediately be suspected. The process of normal breathing should be accomplished with minimal effort. If an individual appears to be using stomach or neck muscles, breathing should be considered labored. These muscles are known as accessory muscles. Infants and young children, however, normally will use abdominal muscles for breathing because they utilize the diaphragm for breathing. A young child or infant who appears to be using their neck or chest muscles to breathe may be experiencing labored breathing.

2. B: The sound of gurgling is indicative of the presence of liquid in the airway. This needs to be cleared immediately because of the risk of aspiration of this liquid into the lungs. Any type of fluid could potentially be in the airway in an emergent situation including saliva, blood, vomit, or secretions. Sometimes log-rolling the patient will help, but when a gurgling sound is heard, suctioning is the best choice for removing the liquid. Suction devices should always be close at hand. These types of devices work by the use of negative pressure through a vacuum pump. Suctioning should be limited to 10 to 15 seconds at a time to prevent interfering with oxygenation. Proper procedure should be followed for handling substances that are suctioned out of the body.

3. A: If trauma is suspected on an unconscious patient, care must be taken to prevent spinal damage. The jaw thrust technique (also known as anterior mandible displacement technique) is the best choice for manually opening the airway. When a patient is unconscious, muscle control of the jaw is suspended, making the jaw easy to open. The index fingers are positioned behind the angle of the jaw, and the jaw is then pushed upward. The tips of the thumbs can be used to keep the jaw in an open position. This allows the head to remain in a neutral position instead of flexed or extended, where damage to the spine could potentially occur.

4. B: There are two types of devices available for establishing and maintaining an airway. The oropharyngeal airway goes into the patient's mouth and helps keep the tongue in the proper position to prevent obstruction. This type of airway may stimulate the gag reflex, which can cause vomiting to occur. This would place the patient at risk for aspiration. If the patient is unconscious, the gag reflex will not be present and this airway can be used. The nasopharyngeal airway utilizes a flexible tube that is inserted through the patient's nostril to establish an airway. This type of airway is less likely to stimulate the gag reflex and is therefore a safer choice for a conscious patient having trouble keeping their airway open. This is also the airway of choice for anyone who is in the active stage of a seizure.

5. B: Mouth-to-mask ventilation is the method that is preferred over other types of ventilation in the field. This is a relatively simple method to perform. The benefit is that both hands are free to make a tight seal around the mouth, enabling the best ventilator volume possible. Mouth-to-mouth ventilation is not a preferred method because of the direct contact with the patient and the inability to protect oneself adequately from body substances. The two-person bag-valve-mask utilizes a self-inflating bag along with a mask. Two EMTs are required to perform this type of ventilation, and the benefit is that 90% to 100% oxygen can be administered when hooked up to an oxygen source. A

one-person valve mask is more difficult to use because one person is required to keep the mask sealed while compressing the bag to deliver oxygen.

6. D: There are many signs that can be observed that would indicate adequate ventilation. A minimum of 12 ventilations per minute is a good indicator, because this means that a breath is being given every 5 seconds, which is the recommended amount. Skin color is also a good indicator. A bluish tinge is indicative of inadequate oxygenation. Gastric distention may indicate the ventilation is occurring too rapidly. Heart rate should return to a normal rate of 60 to 100 beats per minute for an adult as oxygen is being delivered. The chest movement should also be monitored for proper rising and falling as if breathing. If the patient has any signs that indicate inadequate ventilation, the seal on the mask should be verified and the jaw can be repositioned to make sure the airway is open. The possibility of an obstruction should be ruled out. Another method of ventilation can be tried if the one being used is not working sufficiently.

7. C: Trauma to the face can result in excessive bleeding and significant swelling. This may make it difficult to easily ventilate a patient. A suctioning device should be nearby to facilitate clearing of any fluid such as blood or vomit from the airway. This is extremely important. Either a nasal or an oral airway can be established depending upon the severity of the injuries and the location. The patient should be repositioned using a jaw thrust but no head tilt due to potential injury to the spinal cord. Only as a last resort should the patient be repositioned using the jaw thrust and head tilt if no other way is available to open the airway. In some extreme cases where facial trauma involves damage to the skull, the airway can be accessed through the cranial cavity. A tracheotomy in the field would not be one of the first considerations to open an airway.

8. A: The presence of dentures in a patient about to be ventilated can cause significant problems. If possible, the patient should keep the dentures inside his or her mouth in order to get a tight mask seal. The dentures help the mouth retain the proper shape. Without teeth in place, the mouth tends to be sunken and caved, making it difficult to get a tight seal thus making it difficult to properly ventilate a patient. If the dentures are loose, broken, or damaged, they should be immediately removed to prevent airway obstruction. The presence of dentures is something that always needs to be considered, especially in elderly patients.

9. D: Baseline vital signs are extremely important when first assessing a patient. The first step in monitoring the patient is to observe trends in vital signs. The respiratory rate is a measure of how fast or slow an individual is breathing. The normal range for an adult is 12 to 20 breaths per minute and will vary for children, but a newborn typically breathes faster at 40 to 60 breaths per minute (bpm); a 3 year old, 25 to 30 bpm; a 5 to 7 year old, 20 to 25 bpm; and a 10 to 15 year old, 15 to 20. The pulse rate is the number of heartbeats in one minute. A normal pulse rate also varies, but for a newborn it is 120 to 160; 3 year old, 80 to 120; 5 to 10 year old, 70 to 115; 15 year old, 70 to 90; and an adult is 60 to 80. Blood pressure is a measure of the force on the arteries in the heart as it relaxes and contracts, and the reading will vary. The 16-year-old in the question has an elevated pulse and respiratory rate and a low blood pressure.

10. B: Stridor is the term that refers to a loud, high-pitched sound that is made during inspiration. It can be indicative of an upper airway obstruction. Grunting refers to the sound that is made when a patient tries to exhale while the glottis is closed thus keeping the alveoli open with the air unable to move. Wheezing refers to a high-pitched sound that is similar to a whistle and is caused by the narrowing of the bronchioles. This is the sound that may be heard if someone is having an asthma

attack. Crowing is also a high-pitched sound made during inspiration, but it tends to be a long sound similar to the sound made with croup.

11. C: Tachypnea is the medical term used for shallow, fast breathing. A normal respiratory rate is somewhere around 12 to 20 breaths per minute for an adult. Breathing faster than 24 breaths per minute is considered tachypnea. Tachypnea can be caused by many different illnesses, including pneumonia, asthma, chronic obstructive pulmonary disease (COPD), chest pain, or pulmonary embolism. Patients who are breathing rapidly should be administered oxygen at a rate of 15 liters/minute. A nonrebreather mask can be used, or in some cases, a nasal cannula may be substituted. Patients who have a history of asthma or COPD may need to use their inhaler as well to help open up the airway.

12. A: This patient has the appearance of classic emphysema. Emphysema is a type of chronic obstructive pulmonary disease (COPD) caused by smoking or chronic exposure to cigarette smoke or other noxious fumes. This disease works to destroy the surface of the alveoli, making it difficult for gas exchange to occur. As a result, the patient must adapt compensatory breathing strategies in order to get enough oxygen. The shape of the patient's chest will change over time to look like a barrel. The patient will also breathe through pursed lips and will appear to be puffing instead of taking normal breaths. Because breathing is difficult, more calories are burned during the process, and these patients tend to have difficulty maintaining or gaining weight. As this disease advances, any type of exertion will be difficult. Inhalers and chronic oxygen use are common. It is important to look for signs of active cigarette smoking while using oxygen, as this is an extremely dangerous situation.

13. D: The most important step in this scenario is to obtain medical authorization. In some cases, inhalers may not be indicated for a patient who is experiencing respiratory distress. It is important to ascertain whether the patient has her own inhaler, and someone else's inhaler should never be substituted. The patient should also be alert and oriented in order to properly use the inhaler. Once authorization has been obtained, the other items that should be checked before administration are the expiration date of the inhaler, ensuring the inhaler is at room temperature in order to give the appropriate dose, and the inhaler should be shaken a few times. The oxygen mask needs to be removed before administering, and as the patient is inhaling slowly, she should be instructed to hold her breath for as long as she is comfortable able to in order to allow the medication to be absorbed into the lungs.

14. B: A bronchodilator is a type of medication that is administered via an inhaler and is administered directly into the lungs through inhalation. This type of medication is called a beta antagonist bronchodilator and helps the bronchioles to dilate or open up in order to improve oxygen exchange. Generic forms of bronchodilators are albuterol, metaproterenol, and isoetharine. Brand names of bronchodilators include Alupent, Proventil, Metaprel, Ventolin, Bronkosol, Brovana, and Foradil. Pulmicort is a type of inhaled steroid that acts as an anti-inflammatory. These are typically prescribed if a patient is using a bronchodilator more than twice a week or if the patient's asthma interferes with normal activities. Other types of inhaled steroids include AeroBid, Flovent, Azmacort, and Alvesco.

15. A: Respiratory distress is a condition that will be frequently seen as an EMT. The very first step that should be taken when treating a patient with breathing difficulty is to administer oxygen. This is typically administered via a nonrebreather mask at 15 liters/minute. After the patient is receiving oxygen, the focused history and physical examination can begin. The questions in the

focused history will follow the acronym OPQRST (onset, provocation, quality of the distress, radiation of pain, severity of distress, time the respiratory distress started). The physical exam will involve taking and recording vital signs. The most important step, however, is the initiation of oxygen therapy because individuals of any age cannot be without oxygen for very long without suffering from irreversible damage.

16. C: The Sellick maneuver is a method of establishing an airway that helps decrease the risk of regurgitation and can be performed on patients without a gag reflex. This procedure helps to reduce the amount of air that enters the stomach, thus reducing gastric distention. The cricoid ring is located just below the Adam's apple. When this area is depressed, the resultant bump is the cricoid ring. When the cricoid ring is depressed posteriorly, the esophagus will collapse without causing harm to the airway. Three EMTs are required to perform this procedure. Two EMTs are needed to operate the bag mask ventilation (BMV), and the third is needed to hold pressure on the cricoid ring. This pressure needs to be maintained until an endotracheal tube is placed.

17. B: Endotracheal intubation is ventilating a patient through the use of an endotracheal tube inserted into the mouth and into the trachea. The tube has an inflatable cuff that is used to create a tightly fitting seal to prevent air leakage from around the tube. It is a way of ventilating a patient that reduces the amount of air that enters the stomach causing gastric distention. There are certain types of patients who would benefit from this type of intubation before they reach the hospital. A patient who has apnea (absence of breathing) is a good candidate. A patient without a gag reflex is also a good candidate as well as any patient who is not able to safely protect their airway. Endotracheal intubation reduces the risk of aspiration of foreign material into the lungs causing infection. It also allows for proper suctioning as needed and for better oxygenation. A patient who is not responsive to painful stimuli would also be a good candidate.

18. D: Advanced airway techniques can expose an EMT to a number of potential infectious diseases, such as HIV or hepatitis, through contact with bodily fluids. To help prevent this from occurring, a mask, eye protection, and gloves should be worn. Before the tube is inserted, the cuff must be checked for air leaks by inflating the cuff then gently squeezing while listening for air escaping. Tubes come in a range of sizes. Most men will need an 8 to 8.5 mm tube, while women will likely need 7 to 8 mm. Having a 7.5 mm tube on hand will cover most all emergencies. A stylus should be placed into the tube to help with placement, because the tube is flexible and it will be difficult to control the tip of the tube without the support of the stylus.

19. B: A laryngoscope is used to visualize the airway. Parts of the laryngoscope include a light, batteries, and two types of blades. The first type of blade is a straight blade called a Miller blade. This blade is used to lift up the epiglottis in order to see the glottis opening and the vocal cords. The second type of blade is a curved blade called the Macintosh blade. This blade is used to lift up the vallecula, which is the space located between the base of the tongue and the epiglottis. In children, a straight blade is typically used, but in adults, it is usually the preference of the practitioner to select the blade to be used during the procedure. Using the laryngoscope to assist with intubation is the best way to perform this procedure.

20. C: One of the most challenging skills to learn is proper placement of an endotracheal tube, and it is one of the most important. If an endotracheal tube is properly inserted, you should be able to hear breath sounds in the lungs and over the epigastric region. If gurgling sounds are heard, this is an indication that the tube is in the esophagus and needs to be immediately corrected, or the patient can die. The cuff should be deflated, the endotracheal tube should be removed, and the

patient should be ventilated to prevent hypoxia. If breath sounds are only audible on one side of the lungs, the tube may be too far down and is likely to be located in the right main stem bronchi. Other ways to check placement include pulse oximetry to monitor oxygen saturation levels.

21. B: Even with proper placement and confirmation, an endotracheal tube can easily become dislodged. Any time the patient is moved, such as during loading or unloading from the ambulance, the patient himself moves his body or head, or the tube is not secured, it is possible for the tube to become dislodged. This can be very dangerous for the patient, because it prevents proper ventilation from occurring and puts the patient at risk for the complications of oxygen deprivation. The tube can be secured using tape, and the patient can also be placed in a cervical collar to help with controlling head movements. Vital signs should be checked after each time the patient is moved.

22. C: There are four main chambers of the heart. The upper chambers of the heart are the right and left atria, and the lower chambers of the heart are the right and left ventricles. Oxygen-poor blood enters the right atrium and then is pumped into the right ventricle. From here, the blood enters into the pulmonary arteries into the lungs to become oxygenated. The blood is then pumped through the pulmonary veins into the left atrium and then into the left ventricle. From here, the oxygen-rich blood is pumped through the aorta to the rest of the body to deliver oxygen. There are many valves located within the heart to prevent blood from backing up. These valves include the tricuspid, bicuspid, aortic, and pulmonary valves. Arteries carry blood away from the heart, and veins carry blood back to the heart.

23. A: The carotid arteries are the major arteries that are located in the neck. The job of the carotid arteries is to supply blood to the brain. They are located on either side of the neck. These arteries can become blocked or narrowed, and this is called carotid stenosis. This occurs when fatty deposits or plaque builds up in the carotid arteries. Stenosis is typically detected when a swooshing type sound is heard over the carotid artery, which is called a bruit. Risk factors for developing carotid stenosis are hypertension, high cholesterol, heart disease, smoking, drug and alcohol abuse, and heredity. Patients with carotid stenosis are at risk for having a stroke or a transient ischemic attack (TIA, also known as a mini stroke). Symptoms to be aware of are blurred vision, confusion, difficulty communicating, weakness on one side of the body, and sensory loss.

24. C: Patient complaints of chest pain and trouble breathing should be taken seriously, because these may be symptoms of an impending heart attack. Other common symptoms include dull, squeezing, or crushing pain in the chest; pain that radiates to the jaw, neck, upper back, or either of the arms; sweating; abnormal pulse rate and blood pressure; nausea; vomiting; or abdominal pain. When you first arrive, high-flow oxygen should immediately be administered to prevent possible tissue damage from lack of oxygen. The patient's airway, breathing, and circulation should be assessed. Baseline vital signs should be obtained and recorded. Because the patient is experiencing chest pain, additional information should be obtained to help assess the situation. These questions include OPQRST (in relation to pain: the onset, provocation, quality, radiation, severity, and time). Also, determine if the patient has a history of heart issues. You should also find out if the patient has a prescription for nitroglycerin, but you should wait until receiving medical clearance before administering.

25. C: Nitroglycerin is the generic name for a medication that is used to dilate blood vessels, thus allowing the workload of the heart to be reduced. It is commonly referred to as nitro. This will typically result in relief from chest pain but may also cause the blood pressure to be decreased. If a

patient's systolic blood pressure (the top number) is greater than 100 mm Hg, nitroglycerin may be administered. The patient's blood pressure in the above question would allow nitroglycerin to be administered and therefore is not a contraindication. If the patient does not have his own personal prescription for nitroglycerin, he should not receive the medication. Additionally, medical authorization for administering nitro must be obtained from a physician before administration. If the patient has used any erectile dysfunction medications such as Cialis, Viagra, or Levitra within the prior 24 hours, nitroglycerin should not be given, because blood vessels may become extremely relaxed and blood pressure may drop dangerously low. Nitro should not be given to children.

26. A: A typical nitroglycerin dose will be 0.3 to 0.4 milligrams (mg). It is available as a sublingual (under the tongue) tablet, spray, or extended-release capsule. A prescription for extended-release capsules can usually be taken orally three to four times per day. Nitroglycerin given via spray or tablet is usually taken on an as-needed or PRN basis and can be taken up to 10 minutes before any activity that will likely cause angina to occur. If medical authorization has been obtained to give a patient nitroglycerin, the expiration date should be verified before giving a dose. Once the bottle has been opened, nitroglycerin tablets will lose their potency once they have been exposed to light and thus may not be as effective. If no prescription is available, talk with the physician to see if an order is indicated. The patient needs to be properly positioned in a sitting or laying position in case hypotension occurs. Vital signs should be monitored after each dose. An EMT may typically assist with up to three doses given three to five minutes apart as needed.

27. B: The American Heart Association defines the chain of survival as a set of critical interventions that need to occur in order to optimize survival in a cardiac arrest situation. These steps can be initiated by a bystander, and the guidelines were revised to try to simplify the steps for nonmedical bystanders. The first step is timing. EMS should be immediately called and alerted to the situation. Cardiopulmonary resuscitation (CPR) should immediately be started, and this step is critical in improving chances of survival. It must be followed closely by defibrillation using an automated external defibrillator (AED). The fourth step is arrival of EMS on the scene where advanced care life support (ACLS) can be provided such as basic life support, cardiac drugs, or breathing assistance. Research has shown that if these steps are performed within eight minutes, the chance of survival is estimated at approximately 20%, and if they are performed within four minutes and an EMT arrives on the scene within eight minutes, the chance of survival is approximately 40%.

28. D: An automated external defibrillator (AED) is most useful in a patient in sudden cardiac arrest (SCA) who is experiencing ventricular fibrillation. This occurs when the ventricles, or lower chambers of the heart, are beating abnormally fast and in an irregular pattern. By using the AED, the delivery of a shock can help regulate the heart's rhythm. An AED can be used on a patient with ventricular tachycardia without a pulse, but if the patient has a pulse, it can cause irreparable damage, such as asystole. Asystole is a lack of heart rhythm that cannot be shocked into a normal rhythm. AEDs are now found in a wide variety of places, including airports, schools, places of business, and hotels. If an SCA occurs, early intervention is critical in achieving survival. AEDs are relatively easy to use and are computerized to provide detailed but simple instructions to ensure proper use.

29. C: The AED can be used immediately if the cardiac arrest was witnessed. An unwitnessed cardiac arrest requires the use of five cycles of CPR, which is approximately two minutes in length. Once the CPR cycles are completed, the AED should be applied. All direct contact with the patient should be stopped while the AED is in use. Shocking should not be continuously applied until a pulse rate is regained. Rather, shocks should be delivered, then the message from the AED should

be noted and may indicate that no shock should be delivered. If additional shocks are needed, authorization should be obtained from the physician.

30. B: Once the initial CPR has been completed and the AED has been attached to the patient's body, the machine is turned on. If the machine gives instruction to shock the patient based on the rhythm analysis, the shock should be delivered. Immediately following the shock, the patient should be checked for the presence of a pulse. If there is a pulse present, next the patient's breathing should be checked. A decision should then be made about whether to provide high-flow oxygen via a nonrebreather mask or to artificially ventilate the patient. If there is no pulse present, CPR should be restarted for two minutes. The AED will then give instructions on whether to give another shock based on rhythm analysis.

31. A: An automated external defibrillator (AED) should never be used in a moving vehicle. It is very dangerous and puts the patient at risk for injury. If you are transporting a patient who goes into cardiac arrest, the ambulance should be immediately stopped. The AED should be attached to the patient's body, initiate rhythm analysis, and deliver the shock if directed by the AED. An additional contraindication to using the AED is the presence of any water, whether it is weather related or on wet clothing. The patient should not be in contact with any metal. Both water and meal will conduct electricity and may shock others who are around the patient or in contact with those materials.

32. C: The medical condition known as shock occurs when there has been a large volume of blood lost. This reduction in blood volume leads to a reduced amount of oxygen being delivered to tissues, but the brain, heart, lungs, and kidneys are especially affected. This is also known as hypoperfusion. The consequences of shock are tissue damage due to oxygen deprivation and an inability to clear waste products from the body. Hypovolemic shock is an overall reduction in blood volume due to conditions such as dehydration, vomiting, or blood loss, while hemorrhagic shock refers to shock caused by excessive bleeding only. Symptoms of shock include paleness due to decreased skin perfusion, cool and clammy feeling skin, changes in mental status, and hypotension. The heart rate increases to try to quickly pump what is left of the blood supply around the body. Once the blood pressure drops, shock has progressed, and death may be imminent.

33. D: Two of the earliest signs of shock are changes in mental status and heart rate. Any change in oxygen flow to the brain can quickly cause mental status changes. The changes may be small or subtle at first, but as reduced oxygenation continues, the changes will be more noticeable. If a patient initially presents as being alert and oriented without any mental status issues but then begins to appear restless, anxious, or combative, this should be an immediate red flag that early shock may be developing. An elevated heart rate is also an early indicator of shock as the heart tries to beat faster to move blood around. The patient may not have outward signs of bleeding but may in fact be bleeding internally. The symptoms should be treated as early shock.

34. B: Beta-blockers are often prescribed for individuals with conditions such as hypertension, congestive heart failure, history of heart attack, or abnormal heart rhythms. The mechanism of action is to block adrenaline from reacting with the body's beta-receptors. This acts to slow the nerve impulses traveling through the heart. This helps the heart to relax and not work as hard to pump the blood and deliver oxygen. If a patient is presenting with shock and is taking beta-blockers, the heart rate may not increase. Increased heart rate is an early sign of shock. A combination of increased heart rate and vasoconstriction helps to maintain blood pressure in the face of excessive blood loss. Beta-blockers may cause the blood pressure to drop and can lead to

severe shock. Types of beta-blockers include atenolol, metoprolol, sotalol, propranolol, and labetalol. It is important to determine this information when treating a patient with possible shock.

35. B: Precautions need to always be taken to protect oneself from direct contact with any bodily substances such as blood or waste products. These precautions include mask, gown, eye protection, and gloves. The next step would be to immediately assess the airway in order to ventilate the patient with high-flow oxygen. This helps to minimize damage to the body due to oxygen deprivation. Standard procedure should be followed in assessing and establishing the airway. The patient may also require suctioning to clear any material such as blood from the airway. The next step should then be to try to stop or control the bleeding to prevent further blood loss. If there are no lower body injuries, the legs may be elevated 8 to 12 inches to try to increase blood flow to the brain. If lower body injuries are present, the patient should be maintained in a neutral position. The patient should also be prevented from losing body heat by covering him or her with a blanket.

36. A: One of the reasons that it is important to maintain body temperature during shock is to help preserve oxygen and energy. As the body temperature drops, the body will begin to shiver, which will use valuable oxygen and energy in the process. This oxygen could be better used for preventing organ and brain damage. This needs to occur even in warm or hot temperatures. Low body temperature is a sign of shock as well as cold, clammy skin. The cool and clammy skin is due the action of epinephrine and norepinephrine, which are secreted by the adrenal gland in response to the stress of losing blood. This causes vasoconstriction to occur.

37. D: Part of an EMT's job is to assess a situation in which bleeding may be involved. Sometimes the bleeding can be so severe that immediate action needs to be taken in order to prevent further blood loss from occurring. It is important to remember to protect yourself from coming in direct contact with any blood. Bright red blood that is spurting from a wound is likely an arterial bleed. These are the most dangerous bleeds, because arterial pressure is high and the amount of blood loss can be significant. The bright red indicates the blood is oxygenated, having recently left the heart. Venous blood is typically dark red and flows steadily from an injury. It is easier to control because the pressure is lower than with an arterial bleed. A capillary bleed will usually be a slow stream of dark red blood that oozes from a wound. These are generally more superficial and heal quickly.

38. C: Using pressure points is one way to help reduce bleeding. Applying pressure to the femoral artery, which is located in the upper leg, can help control bleeding in a patient with a leg wound. Concentrated direct pressure is another way to help reduce bleeding by applying direct pressure just above the origin of bleeding. Diffuse direct pressure uses the whole hand to apply pressure using gauze to the area where the bleeding is occurring. Wounds that are considered gaping should be packed with sterile gauze. Elevating an extremity above the level of the heart is also useful in reducing or stopping bleeding. If the extremity has any signs of swelling, pain, or obvious fracture, it should not be raised.

39. B: The use of a tourniquet is considered a last resort when other methods for controlling bleeding have failed. Using a tourniquet often will cause permanent and serious damage to surrounding muscles, tissue, nerves, and blood vessels. The majority of the time, amputation will result if a tourniquet is used. If the decision to use a tourniquet has been carefully made, a wide tourniquet should be used instead of an item such as a belt, piece of rope, or a wire. The key is to provide continuous pressure around the entire perimeter of the injury. It should not be placed directly on a joint but rather as close to the bleeding site as is possible. It is imperative that the

tourniquet not be removed after it has been applied because blood clots could potentially mobilize and head to the lungs, causing a pulmonary embolism and possibly death. The use of the tourniquet should be documented carefully and communicated with anyone who may be caring for the patient.

40. C: Blood that is related to a gastrointestinal bleed can provide a lot of information based just on appearance. Blood that appears to be oozing from the mouth, vagina, or rectum may be indicative of internal bleeding and should not be ignored. If the blood is originating from the GI tract, the color, smell, amount of blood, and any other distinguishing characteristics can provide a clue to the source of the bleed. Bright red blood mixed with vomit may be indicative of a new bleeding site. If the vomit is mixed with what appears to be a brownish liquid that looks like coffee grounds, it may be indicative of an older bleed that has been partially digested. This would contain digestive juices as well as the by-products of blood. If there is bleeding occurring lower in the GI tract, such as the small or large intestine, it will appear as black, tarry-looking stools. The blood has gone through the digestive process.

41. A: The first step in any emergency situation is to ensure a patent airway. If a patient is also experiencing excessive bleeding, high-flow oxygen should be initiated to help prevent damage from oxygen deprivation. The patient should immediately be assessed for signs of shock. If the injury is internal bleeding is from a location on the extremity, direct pressure should be applied, followed by a splint. If the bleeding is likely due to an abdominal injury, a pneumatic antishock (PASG) garment may be required. This device should only be applied to patients who have suspected abdominal injuries without injury to the chest area, and the device should only be inflated under the medical direction of a physician. This type of device may provide delay bleeding long enough to arrive at the hospital for treatment. The main goal should be to transport the patient as soon as possible.

42. D: An elderly patient may exhibit atypical symptoms of an acute myocardial infarction (MI) or heart attack. The usual symptoms would involve chest pain, pain radiating in the left arm or jaw or numbness, and profuse sweating. Elderly patients may exhibit some of the normal symptoms. In an elderly patient, chest pain may not be observed. Older patients may instead present with shortness of breath. Other symptoms to be aware of are feeling dizzy, fainting or syncope, pain in the abdominal area, or feeling extremely tired. It is important to remember that the likelihood of cardiac conditions increases with age due to narrowing or stenosis of the arteries. Angina is a common condition in the elderly and is typically managed with nitroglycerin, but symptoms of angina are shortness of breath or chest pain. The elderly also experience changes in circulation when standing up quickly, which can cause dizziness or fainting. This is called syncope and is much more dangerous in the elderly.

43. C: Labor consists of three stages. The first stage starts with contractions that help to propel the baby closer to the birth canal. Initially, the contractions can be abnormal and far apart, but as labor progresses, the contractions will be closer together. The cervix dilates and is measured in centimeters to gauge how far along the first stage of labor is. Contractions help to prepare the cervix, and the presence of bloody show can be seen during this phase. Ten centimeters is the dilation needed to attain in order for the baby's head to fit through the birth canal. A woman enters the second stage of labor as the baby's head enters the birth canal and can be seen through the vaginal opening. This is known as crowning. When this is observed, it is an indication that the baby will be born very quickly and on the scene. The third stage of labor is the afterbirth where the placenta is delivered.

44. B: Once a woman has reached the second stage of labor and crowning is evident, delivery will usually occur fairly quickly. The urge to have a bowel movement may be caused by the feeling of pressure in the lower abdominal area as the baby's head presses against the rectal area. There is a chance that the baby could be born while the mother is trying to move her bowels, so it is best to advise against this. Since delivery is imminent, communication should be occurring with the hospital physician to help guide you through the delivery process.

45. A: Vaginal bleeding that occurs late in pregnancy is usually related to an issue with the placenta. If bleeding is accompanied by severe abdominal pain in the lower abdominal region, it may be due to placental abruption, in which the placenta separates from the uterine wall. Any amount of placental separation from the uterine wall occurs in about 1 out of 150 live births. Placenta previa can also be a possibility where the placenta is positioned low in the uterus and may sometimes cover the cervical opening. As the cervix begins to thin as pregnancy progresses, it may cause bleeding. Any bleeding late in pregnancy can be dangerous. The patient should be treated for the symptoms she is showing. Because of the bleeding and potential for complications, advanced life support (ALS) should be called to assist. Oxygen should be administered through a nonrebreather mask, she should be positioned on her left side to relieve pressure on the vena cava, and the patient should be observed for signs of shock.

46. B: The average length of labor for first-time mothers is 12 to 18 hours. This can vary widely though and is unique to each mother. The length of labor tends to decrease with each subsequent baby. There are many questions that need to be asked of a woman in labor to help assess the situation. The due date is important as well as if there are any known issues with the pregnancy, such as breech position or participation in prenatal care. Information regarding timing of contractions and degree of pain should be obtained. The presence of bleeding or any type of discharge is important to note. The mother should be questioned about the type of pressure she is feeling in her abdominal area as well as if she is feeling the urge to start pushing. All of this information coupled with whether the baby's head is crowning will help in the decision making regarding the possibility of hospital transport.

47. D: If it appears likely that a baby is going to be born imminently without time to get to the hospital, there are steps to take to get ready for the birth. First, all precautions should be taken to avoid contact with any bodily fluid. Next, a sterile field should be set up, utilizing sterile towels or a sterile paper barrier around the lower part of the woman's body. As crowning occurs, it is important NOT to press on the baby's fontanelles, as this is the area that allows for brain growth during the infant's first year. The amniotic sac should be punctured if it is still intact at this point in the delivery. It is extremely important to look at the position of the umbilical cord. If it is wrapped around the baby's neck, attempts should be made to loosen and remove it prior to delivery. If this is not possible, clamp the cord in two places, and then cut the cord to remove the danger.

48. C: Most of the time, a baby is delivered with his or her head facing down. The mouth should be suctioned for any material that may be present, followed by suctioning of the nose. As the head is delivered, the head and body are turned in order for the shoulders to be delivered next. One shoulder is delivered at a time, being very careful in moving the baby's head to assist in the delivery. Once the shoulders are through, the trunk is delivered, while providing good support to the head. The feet are the last to be delivered. The baby needs to be gripped very securely to prevent slipping or dropping. The baby should immediately be wrapped in a warm blanket and kept near the mother's vaginal area to help keep blood from backing up through the umbilical cord into

the placenta. One EMT will continue to care for the mother, while the second EMT will care for the baby. Two clamps need to be placed on the cord. The cord should be tied off and then cut.

49. A: Contractions will continue after the baby is born in order for the placenta to be delivered. The woman will need to push again to expel this material. The umbilical cord should not be pulled as a means of delivering the placenta quicker. This stage of labor may take up to 30 minutes. Once the placenta is delivered, it should be wrapped in a towel and placed in a plastic bag. It should not be discarded, as it needs to be checked to make sure the whole placenta was delivered. If pieces are left inside attached to the uterine wall, infection or excessive bleeding may occur. It is normal for a woman to lose up to 500 milliliters of blood following delivery. More than this is considered excessive. The uterus should be manually massaged if this occurs to try to curb the bleeding. Breast-feeding may also help.

50. B: The APGAR scoring system is a way of concretely assessing an infant's condition upon delivery. Immediately after birth, the infant should be dried with a clean towel and wrapped in a blanket to prevent loss of body temperature. Suctioning should be done as needed to clear material from the mouth and nose. The APGARAPGARAPGAR score should be checked first at 1 minute of life then reassessed at 5 minutes of life. APGAR is an acronym for appearance (coloring of skin), pulse (heart rate), grimace (irritability), activity (muscle tone), and respiratory effort. These areas are each assigned a score between 0 and 2, for a total APGAR score of 10. A score of 2 in a category would indicate the infant meets all criteria. For example, a pulse rate of more than 100 beats per minute would score a 2 because it indicates a good, strong heartbeat.

51. D: Newborn infants should begin breathing on their own within a few seconds after birth. If the infant does not immediately begin to breathe, the infant should be gently rubbed in a circular motion on the back to stimulate breathing. Alternately, you can rub or gently tap on the bottom of the infant's feet. If neither of these tactics works, the next step is to provide positive pressure ventilations at a rate of 30 to 60 per minute. When assessing the heart rate, if it is less than 100 beats per minute, ventilations should be given at a rate of 60 per minute. If the heart rate is less than 80, this indicates a need for chest compressions. There are special standards for conducting CPR on a newborn, and these guidelines should be followed. The infant should be reassessed in 30 seconds. Once the heart rate is above 100, free-flow oxygen should be administered by holding the oxygen mask close to the baby's mouth but not placing it directly on the face.

52. A: A prolapsed cord is an emergent situation that needs to be immediately dealt with. This occurs when the umbilical cord is delivered before the baby. The umbilical cord can be sandwiched between the baby's head and the birth canal and can cut off the oxygen supply to the baby. The umbilical cord should never be cut or pushed back into the birth canal. The mother should be positioned in a way that her head is lower than her feet. The pelvis should be slightly elevated if possible. This helps to relieve pressure on the cord. The mother should receive high-flow oxygen through a nonrebreather mask. Sterile gloves should be used, and two or three fingers can be put into the vagina to try to gently push the baby off the cord. If there is any portion of the umbilical cord outside the birth canal, it should be covered with damp, sterile dressings to prevent the cord from drying out. Immediate transport to a hospital is essential.

53. C: Any infant born before the 37th week of gestation is considered to be premature. Infants are also considered at risk if they are born at a low birth weight of less than 5.5 pounds or 2.5 kg. Babies born prematurely have not had enough time to fully mature the various systems such as cardiac, respiratory, gastrointestinal, and immune. During the last trimester, the baby will gain the

majority of weight. If the baby is born early, it will miss out on adding body weight. Because of the lack of body fat, premature infants will lose body heat very quickly and should be immediately dried and wrapped in blankets to prevent hypothermia from developing. Hypothermia can cause many medical issues in the newborn, including hypoxia or respiratory issues. Not all premature babies will require resuscitation, but if the infant appears to need resuscitation, every effort should be made to do this. Free-flow oxygen should be provided right away, and the baby should be transported to the hospital as soon as possible.

54. D: If a child of any age is in need of oxygen, then the best way to administer it should be determined. Many young children will not allow masks to be placed over their faces because it brings about a fear of suffocation or nor being able to breathe. An oxygen mask should never be forced onto the face of anyone, especially not a child. There are alternatives available for administering oxygen without the use of a mask. Blow-by oxygen involves using a mask but placing it near the mouth and nose without touching. The parents are generally helpful in holding the apparatus while simultaneously calming the child. As long as the child is not in severe respiratory distress, this method should be sufficient in delivering oxygen.

55. B: Obstruction of the airway is a dangerous situation. The obstruction can be complete or partial. If the airway is completely blocked, the child will not be able to speak and will become cyanotic (blue). In a child, back blows are not performed. Back blows can be performed on an infant if the infant is held in the facedown position while supporting the head and neck. In an older child, a finger sweep can be done if the foreign object is seen in the airway. If no foreign objects are seen, abdominal thrusts can be performed. If the child is unresponsive, it is important to try to ventilate the child as you are trying to locate the foreign object.

56. A: Seizures are a very common condition frequently seen by EMTs responding to 911 calls. Seizures in children can be chronic or acute and can be caused by a myriad of reasons including high fever, hypoglycemia, ingestion of poison, or some other cause. The cause of the seizure is not important in the beginning. The most important goal is to prevent injury. Seizures can sometimes evolve into convulsions. After checking to see if the airway is patent, keep the child safe from injury. Nothing should be put in the child's mouth. After the seizure is complete, the child should be positioned in the recovery position, and oxygen should be administered. Antiseizure medication is only given under medical supervision and if the child has a prolonged seizure of greater than 10 minutes in length. If this occurs, ALS assistance will be required.

57. C: Drowning is another condition that is frequently encountered. It is the third cause of death in children up to the age of 14. Drowning by definition is someone who dies from suffocation within 24 hours of being under water for a prolonged period. Near-drowning is someone who survives longer than 24 hours after being under water for a prolonged period. The main goal in a drowning situation is to immobilize the patient if spinal trauma is suspected. In many cases, this will be an unknown and should be done as a precaution. Oftentimes you will arrive, and the patient will already be out of the water. If you arrive and the patient is still in the process of being rescued from the water, it is best not to try a water rescue unless specialized training has been completed. Once the patient is pulled from the water and immobilized, oxygen should be provided. The patient may need to be suctioned. If the patient is unresponsive, chest compressions may be indicated.

58. A: Any burn injury less than three inches in diameter and consisting of first- or second-degree injury is considered a minor burn. Proper treatment would be to first cool the burn by running it under cool water. Ice should never be applied to a burn injury. Wet dressings should also be

avoided. Dry, sterile gauze is the dressing of choice. Fluffy dressings should also be avoided, as the cotton lint may get into the wound. Over-the-counter pain medication may be administered with medical approval. This type of burn may not require transport, and these wounds may heal quickly on their own.

59. B: Shaken baby syndrome is an extreme form of child abuse. This can occur when a caregiver becomes angry and shakes the infant violently to stop the crying or irritable behavior. The infant's brain bounces around inside the skull, causing cerebral contusions. The brain swells and sometimes bleeds. Shaking a baby or any child can lead to permanent brain damage and even death. Symptoms of shaken baby syndrome can range from seizures to changes in behavior, such as irritability or lethargy. The infant may have difficulty breathing, the skin may be cyanotic, and vomiting may occur. The infant may not wake at normal intervals to eat. There may not be obvious physical signs of abuse. There may be fractures evident on x-ray or bleeding behind the eyes. The infant must be carefully cared for in case of spinal injury. Proper authorities must be notified in situations like this.

60. D: The first concern of an EMT is always the medical care of the patient. In this case, it is assessing the signs and symptoms the child is displaying and addressing them appropriately. Transport to a medical facility should occur as soon as possible. Any information conveyed should be objective in nature, stating vital signs, symptoms present, and medical treatment administered. The parents or caregiver should not be accused of child abuse while treating the patient. This will cause appropriate treatment to be delayed and may cause additional injuries. Once the child arrives at the emergency room and care of the child has been transferred, appropriate steps must be followed in starting the reporting process. This process is different in every state. The report will usually include information regarding what you saw at the scene, comments made by the people who were there, and any other pertinent objective information.

61. C: A tracheostomy is a surgical opening in the neck and into the trachea to allow for breathing. A tracheotomy is the surgical procedure to create this opening. A tracheostomy is needed for certain patients to help with breathing with a ventilator over the long term. Many pediatric patients have tracheotomies and live at home with the parents providing care for them. The parents become well versed in taking care of the tracheostomy tube, but occasionally the tube becomes dislodged and needs to be reinserted at the hospital. If the child is unable to breathe in the interim, the EMT may need to help ventilate the patient until admission to the hospital. The first choice is to cover the stoma or opening in the neck. The bag-valve-mask should be placed over the mouth and nose, and the patient can be ventilated. If this is not possible, the second choice would be to ventilate using a smaller mask over the stoma while keeping the patient's mouth closed.

62. A: It is very likely that when an EMT is responding to a situation involving a child, the parents or family will react emotionally. It is important to remember that a professional and caring demeanor must be maintained at all times while trying to treat the child. Any interaction with the family should be calm and supportive. A rule of thumb to remember is that if the parents remain calm, the child will likely remain calm. If the parents are agitated or hysterical, the child may react the same way. Help to calm the parents' anxiety by explaining what is happening and provide reassurance. It is important to refrain from making any promises to the parents about whether their child will be alright. Providing tips on calming down, such as deep breathing, can be helpful. Parents can be useful in administering oxygen and helping to keep the child calm, but it is important to remember not to separate the child from the parents or family unless medically necessary.

63. C: Hypoglycemia means low blood sugar or a blood sugar reading that is less than 70 mg/dL. This happens when too much insulin is in the blood or too little glucose is available. If a person has diabetes, hypoglycemia can occur if a meal is skipped, during illness, or from an increase in exercise without increasing food intake. Symptoms of hypoglycemia can include sweating, hunger, headache, rapid heartbeat, irritability, confusion, or disorientation. Hypoglycemia can progress into seizures, convulsions, fainting, or a coma. It is important to recognize symptoms of hypoglycemia. It may not always be known if someone being treated has diabetes, and the patient may not be wearing a Medic Alert bracelet. Hyperglycemia means high blood sugar. The symptoms of hyperglycemia are frequent urination, increased thirst and hunger, weight loss, tingling in the feet, cuts that don't heal well, feeling tired, and sugar in the urine. The blood glucose level is typically greater than 180 mg/dL.

64. B: The most important treatment for a patient experiencing hypoglycemia is to raise the blood sugar level. As an EMT, oral glucose is the most appropriate treatment. One tube of oral glucose contains 15 grams of sugar in the form of dextrose. It is premeasured and is easier to swallow than oral glucose tablets. The trade names for oral glucose gel are Insta-Glucose and Glutose 15. After the glucose gel is given, the blood sugar should be rechecked in 15 minutes. It is important not to over treat, as this can then cause hyperglycemia. Glucagon is used for hypoglycemia as well but is typically used for profound hypoglycemia with loss of consciousness. Epinephrine is not used in the treatment of hypoglycemia. Orange juice can be used in home treatment of hypoglycemia, but the dose is 4 ounces to provide 15 grams of carbohydrate or sugar.

65. A: There are many different medications used for treating diabetes. Insulin is an injectable medication that requires refrigeration. There are many different schedules that a person with diabetes has, such as the number of injections per day as well as the types of insulin. There are rapid-, short-, intermediate-, and long-acting insulins available. The prescription is individual to the patient based on various factors such as age, lifestyle, and the body's response. There are also oral diabetes medications. There are many different categories of medications, including sulfonylureas (Glucotrol, Diabinese, Orinase, Tolinase), biguanides (Glucophage, Fortamet, Glumetza), and meglitinides (Starlix). There are many, many other types of diabetes medications. It is important to remember that alcohol should not be used with oral diabetes medications or in people with diabetes, as it effects how blood glucose is regulated. For example, hypoglycemia can occur immediately after ingesting alcohol while on oral diabetes medications, and the effects may last up to 12 hours afterward. The symptoms of hypoglycemia and drunkenness are very similar.

66. D: Most allergic reactions have common symptoms. These symptoms on the skin may include hives, itching or pruritus, rash, or flushing in the face. Symptoms may also include respiratory signs, including difficulty breathing, wheezing, coughing, stridor, and tightness in the chest. Swelling may occur anywhere, but common areas are the face, tongue, hands, and feet. The throat may also swell, causing difficulty swallowing. Blood pressure may be low, and the heart may respond by increasing the heart rate in order to maintain blood pressure. Nausea, vomiting, and diarrhea as well as abdominal cramping can also be seen. A severe allergic reaction is called anaphylaxis.

67. B: Epinephrine (also known as adrenalin) is an injectable drug used to treat severe allergic reactions or anaphylaxis. The brand names are EpiPen or Twinject. The mechanism of action is to stimulate the heart, increase blood pressure, and reverse any swelling that may be occurring as a result of the allergy. There can be side effects associated with epinephrine, such as a pounding heartbeat, nausea, vomiting, anxiety, or headache. It is important to note what other medications a patient may be taking, such as beta-blockers, antiarrhythmics, digoxin, MAO inhibitors, or thyroid

medications. Norepinephrine is similar but is used mainly to increase blood pressure in a trauma-type situation. Fexofenadine is used to relieve allergy symptoms, and fluticasone is a synthetic glucocorticoid.

68. D: When evaluating an unconscious patient, it is important to look for clues as to the reason for unconsciousness. Poisoning or overdose is always a possibility. One type of clue to look for is an unusual odor or scent, especially on the patient's breath. The odor of petroleum or garlic could indicate ingestion of certain types of pesticides. The odor of bitter almonds could indicate cyanide poisoning. Other clues to look for would be indicative of a chemical-type burn or strange colors around the patient's mouth. Some poisoning is intentional, as in a suicide attempt, and other types of poisoning are accidental. Children are at high risk for poisoning due to their curious nature. Some poisons will induce vomiting or other abdominal issues right away, but this is not always the case. Most poisons will cause a change in mental status.

69. B: Inhaled toxins can be very dangerous. Because the toxins enter the body through the lungs, absorption is very quick and can lead to poisoning throughout the body. The lining of the airway can be burned by the toxins, and this can lead to difficulty breathing, coughing, and closing of the throat due to swelling. Effects can also include headaches, feeling dizzy, fainting, seizures, and changed mental status. When you encounter a situation that involves inhaled toxins, you immediately should be concerned with potential effects on others in the area. The poison or toxin can still be present in the air. In the case of carbon monoxide, it will not be able to be detected, since it is colorless and odorless. If training has been completed on the use of a self-contained breathing apparatus (SCBA), this should immediately be employed. Otherwise, you will need to wait for specially trained responders. The main goal in initial treatment is to prevent a quick deterioration. The airway should be established and oxygen administered.

70. C: Activated charcoal is one of the main interventions for the management of poison ingestion. The trade names include Actidose, Liqui-Char, and Insta-Char. Activated charcoal is orally administered under medical direction. The mechanism of action is to bind the toxin or poison in the stomach to prevent absorption from occurring. It only works on ingested toxins and not inhaled, injected, or other routes. Activated charcoal should not be used if a patient has ingested either an acid or an alkali substance. It should also be avoided in patients who are unable to swallow or who have a decreased mental status. If a patient receives the activated charcoal early in the course, the outcome is significantly improved. Activated charcoal may cause vomiting, and the dose may need to be given again for optimal effectiveness. The adult dose is usually 25 to 50 grams, while the dose for a child is 12.5 to 25 grams.

71. A: There are three stages to hypothermia. First the patient is alert and oriented, second the patient is becoming disoriented and unresponsive, and third the patient is unresponsive. Vital signs begin to change drastically as the body tries to adapt to declining body temperature. Hypothermic patients may act like they are drunk, and in fact alcohol can worsen the effects of hypothermia. The patient's ability to make decisions may be clouded by both the hypothermia as well as alcohol. The main goal of treatment is to begin to raise the body temperature. This can be done by covering the patient with blankets and placing heat packs warmed to a temperature of 102 to 104° F at strategic places around the body. Oxygen should ideally be administered in a humidified, warm form. These warming steps will not cure the patient but will prevent further heat loss from occurring. The patient should not be allowed to walk because of the possibility of irregular heart rhythms that could potentially be fatal.

72. B: Cold injuries are sometimes called frostbite or frostnip by laypeople. These terms are generally avoided by medical personnel because of the potential for confusion. Local cold injury occurs when there is a decrease in blood flow to an extremity, such as a hand or foot. The body part will experience freezing. Early signs of local cold injury are tingling in the area involved, decreased sensation in this area, and pale skin. As the injury progresses, the skin will turn white and appear waxy, there may be blistering present, and sensation has been lost. The main goal of treatment is to try to gently warm the skin. This will be painful as it occurs. For a long transport, the best option is to place the hand in water warmed to 102 to 104 °F. It is important not to use heat packs or rub or massage the skin. Warm, wet dressings are also contraindicated.

73. D: Hyperthermia is the correct term to describe the condition in which a person's body temperature exceeds 98.6 °F. Heat stroke and heat exhaustion are terms used by many people, but there is considerable confusion surrounding the exact meaning of these terms. It is easier for a body to warm itself up than it is to cool down. Hyperthermia can occur in hot and humid weather. Dehydration compounds the situation. The body relies on radiation and evaporation as a means of cooling, and these mechanisms are impaired in dehydration. Symptoms of hyperthermia include muscle cramps and weakness, feeling dizzy, fainting, and decreased mental status. There can also be nausea, vomiting, and stomach cramping. The primary goal of treatment is to try to cool the patient. An air-conditioned area is helpful, or fanning the can be done to the patient if needed. Oxygen should be provided. If the skin is hot to the touch, ice packs should be placed on the armpits, neck, and groin area. It is helpful to keep the skin wet.

74. D: Elder abuse is an important issue in our country. There are three types of elder abuse—domestic, institutional, and self-neglect. Domestic abuse is maltreatment of an elderly person by the caregiver. Abuse can be physical, sexual, psychological, or in the form of neglect by either the person or the caregiver. It can also involve financial exploitation. Signs of physical abuse in an elderly person may include evidence of injuries in various states of healing, fractures, wounds, or indications that the person has been restrained. Laboratory tests may reveal excessive drug levels or the absence of prescribed drugs in the system. The caregiver may often refuse to leave the patient alone with medical personnel. If any form of abuse is suspected, it imperative to report it to Elder Protective Services. Laws vary from state to state, but EMS are generally mandated to report such issues.

75. C: When dealing with any type of potential psychotic episode or other psychological crisis, it is important to keep yourself safe from possible harm. Information can be obtained from family or those present prior to entering the place where the patient is. Once inside, it is important to take a quick survey of the area. Objects that can be used as potential weapons should be noted and possibly removed. It is important to remember that the EMS team's own equipment, such as scissors or flashlights, can be used as weapons. The patient should not be allowed to block the path to an exit, and the EMS should be near an exit. Body language, such as clenched fists, swearing, or getting physically close to you, can provide clues to behavior or state of mind. If the scene is unsafe or you fear for your own safety, law enforcement should be called to assist before intervening.

76. A: Documentation is one of the most important steps in the restraint process. Documentation must occur before restraints are placed, and then assessment needs to occur every few minutes. Patients who require restraints may be in a state of mind where they blame injuries that occur on the restraints. Only soft leather or cloth restraints should be used, as metal can cause injury. The patient should never be positioned facedown while wearing restraints due to the risk of suffocation. The airway must be easily accessible at all times. If a patient is attempting to bite, a surgical mask or

oxygen mask may be used over the patient's mouth. The laws on restraint use vary from state to state, so it is important to know the law. Sometimes restraints must be applied with law enforcement assistance or under medical guidance. Monitoring of vital signs should continue to ensure the patient's well-being.

77. D: He likely sustained a closed crush injury. This type of injury occurs when extreme force is placed on an area of the body. The injury is inside and does not openly bleed externally. There may be internal bleeding, and shock is a possibility. An open crush injury would involve soft tissue damage and possible damage to internal organs. The wound is open and can be seen with the eye. A laceration is a cut in the skin. The width and depth can vary. An abrasion is a type of scrape that occurs that typically involves the epidermal layer of skin. The wound is superficial but can be very painful. A contusion is another term for a bruise where there is damage to the soft tissue. An avulsion is when part of the tissue is torn off the body. An amputation is when a body part is physically separated from the body. Massive bleeding may occur in the setting of an accidental amputation.

78. B: There are three layers of skin: epidermis, dermis, and subcutaneous or hypodermis. The epidermis is the outermost layer of skin. The dermis continually regenerates and serves as an overall protective barrier to the body. Injuries to this layer are usually superficial and heal quickly. The epidermal layer will gradually begin to thin during the aging process. The dermis is the middle layer. The dermis contains the blood vessels, nerve endings, sweat glands, and oil-secreting glands. If a skin injury occurs in this layer, pain will result. The third layer is the subcutaneous layer, where fat deposition occurs. An injury to this layer will have even more pain and bleeding.

79. A: A patient impaled with any object needs special care. If at all possible, the impaled object should be left in unless it would interfere with medical care such as chest compressions or airway management. The patient may experience significant blood loss if an impaled object is removed on the scene. The main goal of treatment is to control the bleeding. Dressings should be piled around the wound and object to try to stabilize it. These dressings should then be taped in place so the object does not move around. Once the injury is stabilized, transport should occur.

80. D: Any injury to the mouth can cause teeth to become dislodged. If after evaluation, there are no other injuries that need attention, care must be directed to the tooth. A tooth that has been knocked out can be gently rinsed off with water, and then it should be placed in either milk, a tooth-saver solution, if available, or in saline. Saliva is also a great way to try to save a tooth. If the patient is cooperative and willing and it is safe to do so, place the tooth in the patient's mouth between the cheek and gum line. This will help prevent bacteria from getting on the tooth and keep it moist. The tooth should never be grasped by the root, as the ligaments will be damaged, and saving the tooth will be unlikely. It should only be handled by the crown.

81. A: A moderate burn is a full-thickness burn that can cover between 1 to 10% of the body surface area in an adult. It is also considered moderate if it is a partial-thickness burn covering up to 30% of the body surface area. Burns that cover a large amount of body surface area should not be cooled using cool water because this increases the risk for hypothermia. Smaller burns can be cooled with cool water. The most important step to remember is to try to keep the patient warm, as there will be an increase in heat loss through the burn. The body will have a difficult time maintaining the appropriate temperature. Jewelry should be removed as well as any clothing that may still be smoldering. Dry sterile dressings should be used to cover the burn. The patient should be transported to a burn center if there is one close by.

82. C: The very first step in treating a patient who has received an electrical burn is to make sure the source of electricity has been turned off and is no longer in contact with the body. This would be a very dangerous situation for the first responder. Once the source of electricity has been removed, the next step is to administer oxygen and watch the patient for signs of respiratory or cardiac arrest. The automated external defibrillator (AED) should be close by in the event that the patient requires defibrillation. As you examine the patient, look for the entrance and exit wounds. It is important to note that the severity of an electrical burn is usually worse than it appears, with much of the injury internal in nature. Muscles, organs, nerves, and blood vessels may have been injured in the burn. The heart is particularly susceptible. Damage may not be completely evident for quite awhile.

83. C: The human body contains 206 bones. The main bones in the leg are the femur, fibula, tibia, and patella with the tarsal, metatarsal, and phalanges located in the feet. The bones in the arms are the humerus, ulna, and radius with the carpals, metacarpals, and phalanges located in the hand. The bones in the chest region include the clavicle, sternum, scapula, thoracic vertebrae, and ribs. The bones located in the head include the cranium and mandible. In the lower abdominal region, the bones include the pelvis, sacrum, and coccyx. The main purposes of the skeletal system are to provide protection to the internal organs and tissues, give form to the body, and facilitate movement.

84. B: Osteoporosis is the most common bone disease, and it is estimated that at least half of women over the age of 50 have this condition. Approximately 20% of men will also have this condition. Osteoporosis is caused by gradual thinning of the bone and loss of bone density. It can be due to a number of reasons including age; lack of calcium, phosphorus, and vitamin D in the diet; genetic predisposition; low body weight; smoking; alcohol use; and lack of physical activity. Postmenopausal women are also at higher risk due to a reduction in estrogen levels. Any individual with osteoporosis is at risk for fractures. In the elderly, even a short fall can cause a fracture.

85. A: Bone injuries in an extremity will require splinting. The first step is to assess the area around the fracture for sensation, pulse, and circulation. It is important to document this, so when the splint is placed, it will be easier to assess the adequacy of the splinting. After the joints have been immobilized, the splint should be applied. The best way is to apply the splint in the position of the original injury. The bone should not be realigned unless the extremity appears cyanotic or you are unable to detect a pulse. If bones are sticking out of the site, they should be left alone. The splint should be padded to make it comfortable for the patient. The injury should always be splinted before transporting the patient unless there are other life-threatening injuries that take precedence over the fracture. These injuries, such as inability to breathe or excessive bleeding, would always take priority over the fracture and splinting process.

86. D: Any patient who may potentially have an injury to the neck or cervical spine needs to be immobilized before transport in order to prevent additional injuries. A cervical collar or cervical spinal immobilization device is placed around the neck. It is typically used in conjunction with a long or short backboard. The correct size collar should be used so it fits the patient appropriately. The base of the collar should be on the patient's chest, and the chin should fit comfortably on the chin rest and should not be able to move. A long spine board or backboard is used to immobilize from the head all the way to the pelvic area and extremities. It is used with patients who are lying down. The short backboard is used for patients who are sitting down. There are several types that include vest-like boards and rigid short boards. Sometimes the long and short boards are used together. Proper use of these devices is essential to prevent further injury.

87. B: It is extremely important to note that even in the absence of pain, a spinal injury may still be present. Any potential spinal cord injury should be immobilized immediately. The patient should be instructed not to try to move at all. When questioning the patient, it is important to position yourself in a way that allows him to see you without turning his head. Questions to ask the patient may include describing any pain, tenderness, or tingling they may be feeling, exactly what happened in the circumstances surrounding the injury, ability to move the fingers and toes, and also to ask him if he is able to tell where you are touching him at the moment. You may ask the patient to grab both your hands and squeeze in order to assess the equality of the strength in each hand. If the patient is unable to respond, document any important details about the accident scene, such as where the patient was located and the position he was found in.

88. C: As the EMS team approaches the scene of an accident, it should be quickly assessed for types of possible injuries. In the case of a diving accident, compression injury to the spine is likely, but it can also occur in motor vehicle accidents and falls. A distraction injury is tearing or stretching of the spinal cord and occurs in hanging situations as well as gunshot wounds to the spinal cord area. Lateral bending injuries are where the head and neck are bent too far to the side beyond what the body is normally capable of. This is also known as whiplash and can occur in motor vehicle accidents where the car was hit from behind. Stabilization and immobilization are key to initiating treatment in these types of cases.

89. A: A patient who is lying on the ground with a possible spinal cord injury may be placed onto the long backboard using the log-roll technique. Another technique that may be used is the suitable lift or carry. A scoop stretcher may also be utilized. This is a stretcher that can be split in half lengthwise down the middle. The blades can be positioned under the patient and can then be brought together and joined. This type of stretcher helps to minimize movement of the patient. Once on the stretcher or long backboard, the patient should be secured using straps across her chest and pelvis. The patient's legs should also be secured and her arms should be crossed over her chest. Head blocks or towel rolls should be placed around the head to help immobilize in addition to the cervical collar.

90. B: When ready to apply the Kendrick Extrication Device (KED), the first step should be to establish cervical spine stabilization using a cervical collar. Next, evaluation of the patient's sensation, distal pulses, and motor function should occur. This needs to be documented appropriately. The KED should then be slid and positioned behind the patient's back so the spine is centered on the KED. The patient should then be appropriately secured using the straps. At this point, he can be transferred to the long backboard if needed, and sensation, distal pulses, and motor function should be reassessed and documented. The airway should be re-evaluated to make sure it has not been compromised during the application of the KED. This is the manufacturer's general procedure for using the KED, and actual technique should follow established policy and procedures of the EMS agency.

91. D: Manufacturer's instructions should be verified on strap use, but EMTs are taught the following basic procedure. Straps are color coded on the KED for simplifying use. There are two head straps, two leg straps, and three chest straps. First, the chest straps are applied in the order of middle and bottom. The thigh or leg straps are secured next. The head is secured, followed by tightening of the top strap. Ensure that the patient is able to breathe properly and that the strap is not too tight. There are a couple of mnemonics that are used: "My Baby Looks Hot Tonight" or "Money Buys Lots of Hot Toys," in which the first letter of each word helps you to remember the

order. The main point to remember is that the head should be secured after the middle to prevent additional injuries from occurring.

92. A: Traumatic head injury or traumatic brain injury are very serious injuries. These are commonly caused by some kind of blow to the head. The brain is jolted inside the head, causing it to collide with the skull bone. Traumatic head injuries can be closed or open. A closed injury does not break the skull, whereas an open injury does. Mild cases can cause a temporary change in brain function, while more severe cases can cause bruising, bleeding, and other long-term complications. Symptoms may not always be apparent right away. They sometimes develop within a few hours to several days. Symptoms to look for include a change in the pupils, headaches, change in mental status or cognition, memory loss, changes in coordination, seizures, changes in speech or vision, and irritability. Leakage of either clear or bloody drainage from the mouth, ears, or nose can also be an indication. Some head injuries will heal, while others may result in permanent brain damage of varying degrees.

93. D: Helmet use is an important safety factor in injury prevention. There are many different types of helmets including bicycle, motorcycle, and sports helmets. When someone wearing a helmet is involved in an accident, a decision must be made as to whether or not to remove the helmet. One of the main reasons to remove a helmet following an accident would be to adequately access the airway if the airway is compromised. If oxygen needs to be administered, the helmet should be removed. Other reasons include cardiac arrest and the need to immobilize the spine. The way the helmet fits is a major factor in whether to remove it. Loose-fitting helmets that allow the freedom to move the head anyway can be dangerous if there is a possible injury to the spinal cord. Tight-fitting helmets restrict head movement and do not always need to be removed.

94. B: Rapid extrication is the quick removal of a patient. There are certain situations that warrant rapid extrication. These include an unsafe scene where there may be danger of a fire or explosion. Another indication would be that the patient is in the way of accessing another patient who is more seriously injured. Rapid extrication should occur if the patient's medical status indicates the need to immediate care, such as cardiac arrest, possible shock, or difficulty breathing. The decision to make a rapid extrication should be based on the urgency of care or safety but not on the preference of the responder. The disadvantages of rapid extrication include the inability to adequately stabilize the spine in case of spinal injury.

95. C: As the patient is being examined for possible injuries, the acronym that is helpful to remember is DCAP-BTLS. This stands for deformity, contusions, abrasion, punctures or penetrations, burns, tenderness, lacerations, and swelling. Each area of the body is examined, typically starting with the head and moving downward to the neck, chest, abdominal region, and lower extremities. This rapid trauma assessment should only take about one to two minutes of your time. If an injury is identified as the assessment is under way, another EMS should address that injury while the trauma assessment is completed.

96. A: The jugular veins are located on both sides of the neck. The jugular veins drain the blood from the head area including the brain, face, and neck and return it to the heart for oxygen. The jugular veins can provide information on central venous pressure. The height and pulsations of these veins can tell how well the heart is keeping up with the demands being placed on it. The right atrium is the exact chamber being affected. If the veins are flat, blood loss is likely. If the veins are distended, this usually means there is an increase in central venous pressure. This can indicate a backup of blood somewhere in the body. Positioning is important. If the patient is sitting upright,

there should not be any noticeable distention. If the patient is positioned in a 30- to 45-degree-angle and distention is present, this is a cause for concern.

97. A: Rules and regulations vary from state to state and also within the local jurisdiction as to what is stocked on an ambulance for medical supplies. Nonmedical supplies also vary. Personal protective equipment is mandated though to help prevent EMS personnel from acquiring communicable diseases. This type of equipment includes gowns, masks, gloves, and eyewear. Ballistic vests are sometimes worn by EMS personnel who may work in more violent or dangerous areas, but use of these vests is usually personal preference. Medical supplies that are usually included on an ambulance are suctioning equipment, splinting supplies, first-aid materials for caring for wounds, childbirth supplies, and a variety of medications including epinephrine, nitroglycerin, and albuterol sulfate. Supplies needed to ventilate the patient are always stocked, along with an automated external defibrillator and cardiac compression equipment. Nonmedical supplies may include binoculars, maps, and emergency routes that have been preplanned for efficiency.

98. D: Safety is extremely important while responding to an emergency call. Many EMS personnel must take defensive driving courses to help with this. It is often difficult to drive an ambulance and try to predict what a motorist will do when being approached by an emergency vehicle. EMS personnel must obey local regulations at all times. Passing a school bus with its red lights flashing is dangerous and should not be attempted due to the safety of the schoolchildren. Paying attention to the weather and road conditions is essential, as the ambulance is top heavy and can tip over very quickly under adverse conditions. Everyone riding in the ambulance should be wearing a seat belt. When approaching an intersection, it is important to stop and proceed only if the intersection is clear. Defensive driving helps to prevent accidents.

99. B: There are four levels of decontamination: sterilization, high, intermediate, and low levels. Sterilization kills all types of microorganisms. Sterilization utilizes steam pressure or soaking in a chemical solution for a specific amount of time. High-level disinfection will kill all microorganisms except for high numbers of bacterial spores. High-level disinfection is achieved with heat through hot water pasteurization or by soaking in a specific type of chemical, such as Cidex. Intermediate-level disinfection will kill most bacteria, including *Mycobacterium tuberculosis*, viruses and fungi but will most kill bacterial spores. A chemical germicide or a bleach solution is used to perform intermediate-level disinfection. Low-level disinfection will destroy most bacteria, viruses, and fungi but will not kill the tuberculosis bacterium. This level is used for general cleaning, where body fluids are not present.

100. C: When helicopter transport is deemed necessary, it is important to make sure a landing zone has been established. The minimum size requirement is 60 feet by 60 feet, and a size of 100 feet by 100 feet is optimal. The landing zone should be free from obstruction or debris. If headlights of cars or trucks are used, they should be turned off as the helicopter begins to land to refrain from blinding the pilot. The corners of the landing zone should be marked with flares or cones or some suitable substitute. Information about surrounding landmarks is helpful to the pilot. When giving directions, using a method called the clock face method where the helicopter is always heading in the direction of 12 o'clock is helpful. One person in the helicopter should always be designated as the communication person and should not be responsible for providing direct emergency care to the patient.

101. C: The guidelines for appropriate air medical transport will vary, but many medical emergencies and trauma cases are now automatically transported by air if conditions permit. Conditions include falls greater than 15 feet, motor vehicle accidents where a rollover is involved or a passenger has been ejected, or a motorcycle accident where the motorcyclist was traveling greater than 10 miles per hour. Many times, patients with a significant burn injury will need to be transported by helicopter to the nearest burn center. Pediatric patients with significant injuries will also require air transport to a qualified pediatric trauma center. Distance is a factor if transport by ambulance will take longer than 15 minutes. Many decisions need to be made and should be made in conjunction with the medical director. Some limitations do exist with air transport, such as weather and maintenance issues.

102. A: The risk of fire is inherent in many accident-type situations involving motor vehicles, hazardous products, electric wires, and other factors. Extinguishing a fire should only be attempted if specialized training has been received. When an EMT arrives on the scene, the area should be surveyed to check for potentially dangerous situations, such as downed power lines or fluids leaking from a car. If a car is noted to be running, the ignition should be turned off. Smoking anywhere in the area should be avoided. Downed power lines should also be avoided due to the risk of electric shock or death. If there is a person inside a car around downed power lines, the person should remain where they are until the power lines have been disconnected.

103. B: First responders should ideally be trained in handling hazardous materials. There is a program available called the First Responder Awareness Level education program that provides training in these situations. It is important to remember that there are many hazardous situations that may occur. One should practice the utmost care and safety practices when approaching a scene. The wind directions should be ascertained and the scene approached upwind. The area should be cordoned off to prevent bystanders from getting too close. Signs to look for with potentially hazardous scene are off-odors, cloud or fog around the area, and fluid leaking. It is very important to remember that just because an off-odor is not detected, there may still be a danger. Many chemicals and gases do not have an odor. Carbon monoxide is one example of such a gas. The first and foremost rule is to maintain personal safety at all times.

104. D: CHEMTREC is a public service agency also known as the Chemical Transportation Emergency Center, a service of the Chemical Manufacturers Association. This agency can provide online advice 24 hours a day, 7 days per week. It should be one of the very first calls that are placed when dealing with a hazardous situation. The phone number is 1 (800) 424-3900 and is free to anyone who uses the service. Another important resource is the use of Material Safety Data Sheets (MSDSs). These information sheets are required for any chemical product in the United States by the Department of Labor. MSDSs must be easily accessible in all businesses or other places where chemicals are used. The *Emergency Response Guidebook* should also be readily available as a reference. OSHA and NFPA have established guidelines for hazardous materials for use by EMS personnel and other public safety workers.

105. D: A multiple casualty situation is one in which there is more than one person requiring emergency medical care. In order to best attend to the situation, a triage method is used. This is where patients are categorized according to their medical needs. There are typically three levels of priority—highest, second, and lowest. One EMT is in charge of triage and generally has the most knowledge and experience in doing this type of assessment. It is helpful to practice a triage situation periodically to keep skills sharp. Patients are quickly assessed, and then a tag is applied in order to start the care process. The highest priority patients are respiratory issues, uncontrolled

bleeding, multiple and severe medical issues, shock, change in mental status, and severe burns with respiratory involvement. Second priorities would involve burns without respiratory compromise, back injuries, and major bone injuries. Lowest priorities would include minor bone injuries, prolonged respiratory arrest, and cardiopulmonary arrest.

106. A: Duty to act is the legal responsibility of an EMT with a contractual agreement to provide service when needed. This is a very complex issue, which varies around the country. In general, the expectation is that if you are getting paid to provide emergency medical care, then you have the duty or obligation to provide care within your scope of practice and training. In contrast, the Good Samaritan law is supposed to provide some protection to those that assist in an emergency but are not legally required to do so and do not have a duty to act. The good Samaritan law is also complex. In some areas of the country, it may apply to rescue workers and those trained to provide CPR. In other areas of the country, it may only apply to nonmedical bystanders. Both of these laws are not federal laws, so it is important to know your legal responsibilities.

107. C: Negligence is an injury that occurs as a direct result of an error or omission by an EMT that is a normal standard of care or practice. The key is deciding what would usually be done in a certain situation by an EMT with similar training and experience. In order for negligence to have occurred, four criteria must be present. The first is duty to act. The EMT must have failed to provide emergency services. The second is breach of duty. The EMT must have failed to provide the appropriate level of service that another EMT would have provided in the same type of case and with similar training, education, and experience. The third is that the patient incurred some type of injury. The last criterion is that the patient incurred this injury as a direct result of the EMT's action or omission. All four of these must be met in order for negligence to be considered.

108. B: Abandonment is when an EMT stops care without proper authorization from the patient, or does not make sure that someone with the same or higher qualifications is taking care of the patient. Once you begin to provide emergency care to a patient, it must continue. It is permissible to transfer the care of the patient to a more trained or specialized EMT, to the care of an emergency room physician, or to some other specialist more qualified to care for the patient. It is not abandonment if you are not able to treat the patient because of an unsafe scene. If the patient declines or refuses treatment for whatever reason, it is not considered abandonment.

109. B: Expressed consent is providing direct confirmation by the patient that treatment can be provided. The patient must be of legal age in order to provide consent. In many states, this is the age that one is considered an adult and is usually around the age of 18. There may be several exceptions to this rule, including a minor who is pregnant, married, or legally emancipated. The person must also be able to make a decision that considers the implications or consequences of proposed treatment. If the patient is mentally incapacitated for any reason, such as dementia or drug or alcohol ingestion, then expressed consent cannot be given. In cases such as this, implied consent may be assumed or may be given by a spouse or other close family member. The other criteria would be that the patient or legal guardian understands the risks and benefits of the proposed treatment. Treatment cannot commence until the criteria have been met.

110. D: Most parents will willingly provide legal consent for treatment for their child. In very rare and unusual situations, consent may not be provided. Sometimes this is not an issue if the injury is not a threat to the child's life. In other circumstances, quick action must be taken. The best course of action in a life-threatening situation would be to summon the help of the police. The officer would be able to take the child into protective custody, and then treatment can begin without issue.

Physically removing a child from the situation could be dangerous for the child, the adults involved in the situation, as well as the EMT responding.

111. A: Adults are legally able to make their own decisions regarding medical care if they are of sound mind. Even if the patient is obviously injured or sick, the patient may refuse treatment. The EMT does not get to decide what is best for the patient, even if it means that the patient's medical condition will get worse without treatment. If an EMT decides to treat a patient who has refused treatment, an assault and battery charge could potentially be filed against the EMT. If the EMT transports the patient without permission or consent, a kidnapping charge could potentially be filed against the EMT. If an adult refuses treatment, the EMTs have a responsibility to make sure the patient knows the consequences. This must be done verbally with the patient. The EMTs must also be sure there is nothing impeding the decision the patient is making, such as drugs or alcohol.

112. C: A mentally competent adult is allowed to refuse treatment. If the patient does not change his mind about accepting treatment, there are several steps that can be taken. One step is contacting the medical director, who may be able to convince the patient to accept treatment and transport. If the patient is planning to harm himself, the police may be called to assist; however, the police cannot force a patient to accept treatment, either. If all options have been exhausted, careful documentation is key in case the patient later decides to take legal action. Documentation should include the assessment, treatment that was offered, how the treatment was explained, and the implications of refusing care. The patient should sign a release from liability form if he is willing. If the patient refuses to sign the form, it is especially important to get a witness who is not part of the EMS to sign the form.

113. D: An advanced directive is a document that specifies the type of care a patient does and does not want in the event she is unable to make her own decisions at a future time. A living will is one type. This document specifies the type of life-sustaining treatment that is acceptable and the level of care in certain situations. There are often degrees of care, such as the number of resuscitation attempts; basic life support; full life support, including any means available to maintain life; or comfort care. Durable power of attorney specifies the guardian who will be able to make decisions for the patient in the event that the patient is not able to make these decisions. A do-not-resuscitate (DNR) order is also a type of advanced directive that is written by a physician under the direction of the patient. This directs the care providers to withhold life-sustaining treatment when cardiac or respiratory arrest occurs. The patient may revoke the advanced directive at any time.

114. B: A patient may have a DNR order on file with their primary care physician and the local hospital. Many times an EMT responding to a call will not have immediate access to this information. If written documentation cannot be produced at the time of cardiac or respiratory arrest, CPR must be initiated. Patients may submit copies of a DNR order to the local EMS in order to help with decision making. Another point to note is that if the patient or the durable power of attorney has second thoughts about life-sustaining treatment at the time treatment is needed, treatment cannot be withheld. It is important to learn the exact local or state guidelines or regulations about providing life-sustaining treatment and the EMS role. These regulations regarding these advanced directives will vary from state to state or county to county.

115. B: All aspects of patient care are considered confidential. This means that the patient has the right to privacy, even if other people are around who are not directly authorized to provide care to the patient. An EMT must be sensitive to this information and not discuss any private information in front of others. The patient must give permission for information to be given to others. There are

exceptions to this rule. When the patient's care is being transferred from the EMS to the hospital, information must be reported. There are many incidents that require police assistance, and information can be divulged in these cases. These include cases of rape, abuse, accidents occurring in the workplace, gunshot wounds, or animal bites. Information can be provided to insurance companies in order for payment to be received, and information can be discussed in court if an EMT is subpoenaed. Care should not be discussed with a neighbor, the media, or anyone else who is not authorized.

116. C: HIPAA is a federal law enacted in 1996. HIPAA stands for the Health Insurance Portability and Accountability Act, and it came into full compliance in 2003. This law is a gray area for EMS systems because medical care is provided out of the hospital or usual healthcare setting. The main point to remember is that individual EMS system policies and procedures should be followed with regards to how this federal law is applied. The law does apply to healthcare providers who electronically bill for medical services. HIPAA deals with privacy issues and helps to protect medical records. It applies directly to health insurance plans, healthcare providers, and healthcare clearinghouses. HIPAA does not override confidentiality laws that are already in place to protect patients. Maintaining patient confidentiality is extremely important in whatever manner it is achieved.

117. A: Many patients have designated themselves as organ donors upon death. This is often indicated on the patient's driver's license or may be indicated on a donor card. A legal document must be available and signed by the organ donor specifying wishes for organ donation. As an EMT, medical care must continue to be provided at the appropriate level, regardless of whether the patient is an organ donor. A wish to donate organs upon death is important, but the wish cannot be honored until death occurs. Unless the patient has a DNR order on record, all life-sustaining treatment should be offered and attempted. If this does not happen, the EMT could potentially be held responsible for negligence. The main concern is always saving the patient's life. The organ donation designation comes second.

118. C: The Medic Alert system is a service that a patient enrolls in to help emergency responders with medical information. The patient may have a card in their wallet, or the EMT may be able to call an 800 number to obtain appropriate information about the patient. Most patients will wear some type of jewelry, such as a bracelet or necklace to indicate their condition. This may include past medical history, past surgeries, allergies, medications, and emergency contact information. Many patients choose this service with conditions such as heart disease, diabetes, severe allergies, or seizure disorders. This type of service is especially helpful if the patient is unresponsive or unable to communicate.

119. D: Oftentimes when an emergency call is made, the scene is also identified as a possible crime scene. The first and foremost concern is EMT safety. The next concern is the emergency treatment of the patient. The EMT should not enter a crime scene unless police have arrived on the scene. Any delays that occur in treating the patient, such as having to wait for police, should be carefully documented. The EMT must take care not to interfere with the crime scene or disturb evidence. The exception would be if the potential evidence is interfering with the emergency treatment of the patient. In the case of a gunshot wound, it is important to try not to destroy the clothing when removing it from the patient, as this may be an important piece of evidence. Documentation of anything the EMT has seen or heard while at the scene is also very important. Any information documented should be objective and factual.

120. A: A needle stick or other sharp injury can be an extremely dangerous situation. Many healthcare workers, including EMTs, are at risk for this type of injury. Exposure to hepatitis B and C as well as HIV/AIDS or other bloodborne pathogens is a possibility. In 1991, the Occupational Safety and Health Administration (OSHA) enacted the Occupational Exposure to Bloodborne Pathogens Standard. It was designed to protect any worker with a risk of exposure to blood or other infectious materials. This calls for Universal Precautions to be practiced in all settings. This is a way to help protect workers by specifying how blood and other fluids are handled and treated. It also spells out how sharps and needles should be safely disposed of. The standards call for the use of personal protective equipment (PPE), such as gowns, masks, gloves, and eyewear. It is important to understand the standards in order to adequately protect oneself from bloodborne infection.

Practice Test #2

Practice Questions

1. You respond to a call for an elderly woman who is experiencing difficulty breathing. While evaluating the patient, you hear gurgling in her airway. You decide to use suction to clear the airway. Which of the following principles do you apply?
    a. Suction for a minimum of 30 seconds
    b. Insert catheter into the bronchi
    c. Follow body substance isolation precautions when suctioning the airway
    d. Any type of catheter will work for suctioning

2. You must measure the patient prior to inserting a suction catheter into the airway. What is the appropriate method for assessing the length of catheter that is safe to insert?
    a. Measure the distance between the corner of the mouth and the larynx
    b. Measure the distance between the corner of the mouth and the angle of the jaw
    c. Measure the distance between the tip of the nose and the earlobe
    d. Measure the distance between the corner of the mouth and the earlobe

3. Which of the following is the structure that acts as a flap to prevent food and liquid from entering the trachea?
    a. Epiglottis
    b. Uvula
    c. Cricoid ring
    d. Diaphragm

4. Your adult patient has a respiratory rate of 20 breaths per minute. Which of the following best describes this respiratory rate?
    a. Slow rate
    b. Normal rate
    c. Inadequate breathing
    d. Fast rate

5. Your patient's respiratory rate is normal, but he is complaining of shortness of breath. You observe that his chest is moving only slightly when he breathes. What do you suspect?
    a. Inadequate tidal volume
    b. Cyanosis
    c. Pneumonia
    d. Bronchitis

6. Which of the following is the most frequently seen symptom of acute respiratory distress?
    a. Cyanosis
    b. Absent breath sounds
    c. Rapid or slow respiratory rate
    d. Change in level of consciousness

7. Which is the most preferable of the four techniques for artificial ventilation?
   a. One-person bag-valve-mask
   b. Mouth-to-mask
   c. Two-person bag-valve-mask
   d. Flow-restricted, oxygen-powered ventilation device

8. You arrive at a multiple vehicle accident where a nonbreathing patient appears to have a cervical spine injury. What do you do to modify your ventilation technique?
   a. Have a second EMT stabilize the patient's head, or use your knees to prevent movement
   b. Use the head tilt to open the airway
   c. Push down on the chin to open the airway
   d. Position yourself over the patient's chest to best observe the respirations

9. When inserting a nasopharyngeal airway, what technique is appropriate?
   a. The correct-size airway would extend from the tip of the nose to the larynx
   b. Lubricate the airway with a petroleum-based lubricant
   c. Insert the airway with the bevel up
   d. Use a water-soluble lubricant

10. You are attempting to ventilate a nonbreathing patient who has a tracheal stoma. If ventilation through the stoma results in air escaping through the mouth and nose, what is your next action?
    a. Suction the stoma
    b. Close the mouth and pinch the nose
    c. Cover the stoma, and ventilate through the mouth
    d. Insert a nasopharyngeal airway

11. When ventilating a trauma patient, what technique is appropriate for opening the airway?
    a. Tracheotomy
    b. Head tilt with jaw thrust
    c. Jaw thrust
    d. Endotracheal tube

12. A full oxygen tank has about 2,000 pounds of pressure per square inch. Which technique for transporting oxygen is appropriate?
    a. Secure tanks to prevent falling and rolling during transport
    b. Wrap tanks with blankets to prevent contact with other tanks
    c. Valves and gauges are the most secure parts of the tanks
    d. Oxygen tanks do not explode, so no special precautions are necessary

13. During your initial assessment of a patient, your general impression takes only a few seconds. While forming your general impression, what is the most important goal?
    a. Diagnose the patient's illness and note the age, gender, and race
    b. Prioritize care, form a plan of action, and establish nature of illness or mechanism of injury
    c. Determine if there are life-threatening injuries
    d. Transport the patient, provide oxygen if needed, and start IV therapy

14. What is meant by the statement, the patient is "oriented times three"?
    a. The patient responds to his name and recognizes his family
    b. The patient responds to his name only
    c. The patient is unable to respond verbally
    d. The patient answers the questions appropriately, "who, where, and when"

15. Which of the following is a nonobservable condition as described by the patient?
    a. Sign
    b. Symptom
    c. Diagnosis
    d. Sensation

16. Capillary refill refers to the amount of time required for blood to return to the capillary bed after applying and releasing pressure to a fingernail. What is a normal capillary refill time?
    a. 5 seconds
    b. 10 seconds
    c. Less than 2 seconds
    d. More than 6 seconds

17. When using directional terminology to describe an injury that is on an extremity, near the trunk, what is the best term?
    a. Distal
    b. Proximal
    c. Posterior
    d. Lateral

18. You have a patient with an open wound on the back. You decide to position the patient in a prone position. What does this position entail?
    a. Lying on the back
    b. Lying on the abdomen
    c. Lying down with the feet elevated
    d. Sitting upright

19. Your patient has injuries to both arms. You decide to check the pulse in the carotid arteries. Where do you find the carotid pulsations?
    a. In the inguinal area
    b. In the axilla
    c. Lateral to the larynx
    d. Posterior lateral neck

20. Which of the following is the normal respiratory rate for an adult?
    a. 25 to 50 BPM
    b. 5 to 10 BPM
    c. 30 to 40 BPM
    d. 12 to 20 BPM

21. When assessing the circulation of the lower extremities, which arteries do you use?
    a. Femoral and popliteal arteries
    b. Internal iliac and brachial arteries
    c. Posterior tibial and dorsalis pedis arteries
    d. External carotid and common iliac arteries

22. What is the preferred nonhospital method of delivery for high-concentration oxygen therapy?
    a. Nasal cannula
    b. Nonrebreather mask
    c. Oxygen tent
    d. Ventilator

23. You arrive at a patient's home, and during your initial assessment you note that the elderly man has a bluish tint to his lips and fingernails and his skin is cool and clammy. What is your **best** response?
    a. Administer oxygen because he is cyanotic
    b. Wrap him in a warm blanket because he is probably just cold
    c. Perform CPR because he may be having a heart attack
    d. Give him a warm drink, and then transport him

24. Which of the following refers to the evaluation of the environment surrounding the patient to ensure your safety before entering that location?
    a. Body substance isolation precautions
    b. Personal precautions
    c. Scene size up
    d. Mechanism of injury

25. You enter the small apartment of a woman who called 911 complaining of a headache and dizziness. Upon entering, you notice that the oven door is open and the gas burners on the stove are set on high. The patient's husband is lying on the couch and states he is not feeling well, either. You suspect carbon monoxide poisoning. What is your initial response?
    a. Remove both patients from the home, and call for additional EMTs for transport
    b. Instruct the husband to wait and another EMT will come shortly to transport him
    c. Administer oxygen, and see if the symptoms subside
    d. Administer oxygen and start IV therapy on both patients, transport the wife, and come back for the husband

26. You respond to a 911 call for a possible gunshot wound patient. You arrive before the police and notice an injured man lying on the street with several men arguing in his vicinity. Which **initial** action is preferable?
    a. Instruct the men to leave so you can treat the patient
    b. Wait for the police to secure the scene, and then proceed
    c. Explain to the bystanders that the police are on their way, and then proceed
    d. Drive slowly into the crowd so you can access the injured person

27. When you perform the rapid trauma assessment, you examine the patient for injuries using the acronym DCAP-BTLS. What does the letter "P" represent?
   a. Pulse
   b. Perfusion
   c. Position of function
   d. Penetrations or punctures

28. You arrive at a multiple-vehicle accident in which one car was T-boned by another car. When you examine a young male driver, you observe that his left arm is severely deformed. What is the most common cause of traumatic deformity of a limb?
   a. Torn ligament
   b. Broken bone
   c. Dislocation
   d. Extensive swelling

29. Which of the following describes a scrape in which the top layers of the skin are missing?
   a. Contusion
   b. Puncture
   c. Laceration
   d. Abrasion

30. When examining the chest of a trauma patient, upon auscultation you hear the sound of bones rubbing against each other. What is the medical term for this sound?
   a. Croup
   b. Wheezing
   c. Crepitation
   d. Gurgling

31. You answer a call for a 14-year-old boy who is complaining of pain in the area of his appendix. When describing this area to another EMT, which of the following terms is accurate?
   a. RUQ
   b. RLQ
   c. LUQ
   d. LLQ

32. When assessing the neck of a trauma patient, the jugular veins may indicate an increase or decrease in circulatory pressure. Which of the following statements regarding the jugular veins is accurate?
   a. Distended jugular veins in a sitting patient signify increased circulatory pressure
   b. Distended jugular veins in a supine patient signify increased circulatory pressure
   c. Flat jugular veins in a sitting patient signify decreased circulatory pressure
   d. Flat jugular veins in a supine patient signify increased circulatory pressure

33. What is the correct term for information you gain from observing and assessing a patient?
   a. Subjective assessment
   b. Rapid assessment
   c. Objective assessment
   d. Patient history

34. On each side of the face there is a structure composed of a slender bar of bone that connects the temporal bone to the cheekbone. What is the medical term for this formation?
   a. Mandible
   b. Maxilla
   c. Orbit
   d. Zygomatic arch

35. How often do you reassess and record the vital signs on a stable patient?
   a. Every 10 minutes
   b. Every 5 minutes
   c. Every 15 minutes
   d. Every 30 minutes

36. You make an error while writing your report of patient care. What is the correct method of correcting the mistake?
   a. Erase and enter the information correctly
   b. Obliterate it completely with heavy pen marks, and then rewrite it
   c. Simply white it out with correction fluid, and then rewrite it
   d. Strike through the error with one horizontal line, and then initial and rewrite it

37. Many patients refer to their medications by the name given by the company that manufactures the drug. What is the term for this name?
   a. Generic name
   b. Trade name
   c. Popular name
   d. Pharmacology name

38. You speak to a physician who instructs you to administer a medication to your patient. What is your immediate response to his order?
   a. Repeat the name, route of administration, and dosage to confirm the order with the physician
   b. Repeat the name, route of administration, and dosage to your partner to confirm the order
   c. Call your supervisor and confirm the order
   d. Call the hospital pharmacist and confirm the order

39. Which of the following conditions is a degenerative disease in which the patient loses alveolar surface area, directly related to extensive exposure to noxious substances such as cigarette smoke?
   a. Asthma
   b. Emphysema
   c. Stridor
   d. Pneumonia

40. What is the medication you would initially administer to a patient in respiratory distress?
   a. Proventil inhaler
   b. Oxygen
   c. Epinephrine
   d. Lasix

41. When the heart does not receive adequate oxygen, the patient may feel pain in the chest, especially following exertion. What is the medical term for this type of pain?
   a. Angina
   b. Dyspnea
   c. Congestive heart failure
   d. Tachycardia

42. What are the major arteries to the brain that are located on either side of the neck?
   a. Temporal
   b. Jugular
   c. Carotid
   d. Popliteal

43. When you assess a patient at a multiple-vehicle accident site, you note that the patient's skin is clammy and pale, her pulse is rapid and weak, and she is complaining of nausea. What do you immediately suspect?
   a. Head injury
   b. Broken bone
   c. Heart attack
   d. Shock

44. You suspect that the patient is in shock (hypoperfusion) based on all the signs and symptoms, but her blood pressure is normal. What is your response?
   a. The B/P drop is the most reliable sign, so you ignore the other symptoms
   b. Because the B/P is frequently a late sign of shock, treat the patient for shock, based on the other signs and symptoms
   c. If the B/P is normal, the patient must be hypothermic
   d. If the B/P is normal, use a warming blanket and hydrate the patient

45. Which of the following is the generic name for a sublingual drug that relieves the symptoms of angina?
   a. Nitroglycerin
   b. Oxygen
   c. Digitalis
   d. Lasix (furosemide)

46. After administering nitroglycerin sublingually, what is the next appropriate step?
   a. Place the patient in Trendelenburg
   b. Measure and record the B/P
   c. Have the patient rinse her mouth with water
   d. Use defibrillation

47. Which primary intervention gives the patient the greatest chance for survival of a cardiac arrest?
   a. IV therapy
   b. Nitroglycerin
   c. Defibrillation
   d. Oxygen administration

48. When a patient experiences stabbing chest pain that increases in severity when taking a deep breath, what is the probable origin of the discomfort?
    a. Circulatory system
    b. GI tract
    c. Gallbladder
    d. Respiratory system

49. You arrive at a patient's home and note that the middle-aged man is pale, sweating, and anxious. He states that he is sure he is going to die, and he says that he feels like an elephant is sitting on his chest. The patient appears to be having difficulty breathing. What do you suspect?
    a. Cardiac arrest
    b. Cardiac compromise
    c. Panic attack
    d. Bleeding ulcer

50. Which of the following situations requires the use of the automatic external defibrillator (AED)?
    a. You are unable to hear the heartbeat, although you can feel a weak carotid pulse
    b. You are unable to hear the heartbeat, and unable to palpate any pulse
    c. The patient is awake, but has a very irregular heart rhythm
    d. The patient is unresponsive, but you note a pedal pulse

51. Which of the following terms refers to a condition in which the heart is "quivering" and not producing a pulse?
    a. Ventricular tachycardia
    b. Atrial tachycardia
    c. Heart block
    d. Fibrillation

52. If a patient has a very *low white blood count*, what is the main health concern?
    a. Anemia
    b. Inability to fight infection
    c. Uncontrolled bleeding
    d. Blood clot formation

53. What do red blood cells deliver to all the tissue of the body?
    a. Hemoglobin
    b. Iron
    c. Oxygen
    d. Plasma

54. What is the medical term that describes a patient who is responding inappropriately, either verbally or nonverbally?
    a. Altered mental status
    b. Seizure
    c. Coma
    d. Hypoglycemia

55. You arrive at a scene where a young man is lying on the floor, breathing, but appearing confused. Bystanders state that the patient had a seizure. What is the appropriate response?
   a. Because the seizure is over, allow the patient to recover and release him
   b. Assess the vital signs, then transport the patient to the ER for further diagnosis
   c. Because seizures are the result of epilepsy, ask him for his medications, administer them, and then release the patient
   d. Seizures are common, so instruct him to see his physician in the near future

56. You respond to a call made by a child stating that her mother is sleeping on the couch and will not wake up. When you arrive, you note that the mother's color is pink, her breath smells "fruity," and her pulse and respirations are within normal ranges, but she does not respond to verbal stimuli. What is your next action?
   a. Check the refrigerator for insulin
   b. Give her orange juice
   c. Start an IV and administer glucose
   d. Start CPR

57. Which category does a patient with a blood glucose level of 80 or below fall within?
   a. Hyperglycemic
   b. Normal range
   c. Hypoglycemic
   d. Diabetic

58. Which of the following statements is inaccurate regarding the administration of oral glucose gel?
   a. Place the tip of the tube between the cheek and the gum
   b. If the patient is unconscious, administer the gel very slowly
   c. Administer oral glucose to any patient with altered mental status
   d. Perform ongoing assessments every five minutes until the patient is stable

59. Which of the following is the most significant sign of hypoperfusion during an allergic reaction?
   a. Rash
   b. Edema
   c. Altered mental state
   d. Wheezing

60. Which term refers to a serious allergic reaction that could be life threatening?
   a. Anaphylaxis
   b. Wheezing
   c. Edema
   d. Rash

61. You respond to a call where a six-year-old boy is experiencing an allergic reaction to a bee sting. Upon arrival, you observe that the child is loudly wheezing and appears to have facial edema. The mother informs you that he has an epinephrine autoinjector pen because of a peanut allergy. What is the appropriate action?
    a. Administer the epinephrine
    b. Call for medical direction
    c. Transport the patient without giving the epinephrine
    d. Have the child administer the epinephrine

62. What is the first treatment for a patient who inhaled a toxin?
    a. Epinephrine
    b. Oxygen
    c. IV therapy
    d. Fresh air

63. You arrive at the home of a snakebite patient. Which of the following actions is inappropriate?
    a. Administer oxygen
    b. Have suction available
    c. Immobilize the affected extremity
    d. Catch the snake for identification

64. Which type of poisoning may require the administration of activated charcoal?
    a. Ingested poison
    b. Absorbed poison
    c. Injected poison
    d. Inhaled poison

65. When treating a patient who is hypothermic, which of the following is inappropriate?
    a. Administer high-flow oxygen
    b. Remove wet clothing and cover the patient with a blanket
    c. Gently massage the extremities
    d. Do not allow the patient to eat or drink stimulants

66. In late-stage hypothermia, what is the skin color?
    a. Red
    b. Pink
    c. Pale, cyanotic
    d. Jaundiced, yellow

67. When you inspect the feet of a homeless man after exposure to extremely cold temperatures, you observe that the skin of his toes is white and waxy and feels frozen on palpitation. What do you suspect?
    a. Superficial injury
    b. No injury
    c. Good prognosis
    d. Deep-tissue damage

68. You arrive at the scene of a twenty-year-old woman who was running in a marathon on a 90º day. The woman's skin is quite red and feels hot to the touch. She appears disoriented. Which of the following treatments is inappropriate?
    a. Place the patient in the air-conditioned ambulance
    b. Apply cool packs to the neck, groin, and axilla
    c. Keep the patient dry
    d. Transport to the hospital immediately

69. You arrive at a large swimming pool where a 14-year-old boy is floating in the water supported by several people. The lifeguard informs you that the boy hit his head on the diving board as he attempted a dive, and he was unable to move after he entered the water. Which action is inappropriate?
    a. Place the boy on a long backboard while he is still in the water
    b. Apply a cervical spine immobilization device
    c. Have the people who are supporting the boy lift him out of the water
    d. Strap the boy onto the long backboard with two or more straps

70. What is the term for the stage of labor in which the head of the baby is bulging from the vaginal orifice?
    a. Crowning
    b. Pushing
    c. Bloody show
    d. Dilation

71. The medical term for an unborn baby who is still developing in the uterus?
    a. Zygote
    b. Fetus
    c. Newborn
    d. Infant

72. Once pulsations in the umbilical cord have stopped, it is time to clamp the cord. What is the proper technique?
    a. Clamp four finger widths from the baby's body, then four to five inches from the first clamp
    b. Clamp close to the baby's body, then another four inches from the first clamp
    c. Attach two clamps four finger widths from the baby's body
    d. Attach one clamp near the baby's body

73. You arrive at the home of a pregnant woman who has gone into late-stage labor. When you assess her, you realize that the baby is crowning, so you prepare to deliver the child. As the head emerges, the umbilical cord is around the baby's neck. What is your next action?
    a. Deliver the baby, and then unwind the cord from the neck
    b. Attempt to remove the cord from the neck; if unable, clamp it in two places and cut between the clamps
    c. Do nothing, transfer the baby to the hospital
    d. Cut the cord, and deliver the baby

74. You successfully deliver a baby in the patient's home. The placenta does not follow within 20 minutes of delivery. Which option is incorrect?
    a. Allow the placenta to deliver on its own
    b. Encourage the mother to push when she has a contraction
    c. Gently pull on the cord
    d. The placenta sometimes takes up to 30 minutes to deliver

75. What is the medical term for the type of delivery in which the buttocks or legs emerge first?
    a. Cephalic
    b. Breech presentation
    c. Prolapsed cord
    d. Premature birth

76. Nearly half of the elderly patients with myocardial infarction (MI) present in the ER with only one complaint. Which symptom of MI is most common in the older patient?
    a. Chest pain
    b. Nausea
    c. Shortness of breath
    d. Numbness in the arm

77. What is the medical term for the pathological syndrome in which there is mental deterioration with resulting loss of the higher functions of the brain?
    a. Syncope
    b. Vertigo
    c. Dementia
    d. TIA

78. Which of the following conditions often presents with emesis that contains black particles that appear like "coffee grounds"?
    a. Bleeding from the colon
    b. Bleeding from the bladder
    c. Bleeding from the respiratory system
    d. Bleeding from the stomach

79. You respond to three separate calls to the same house where an elderly man lives with his son. Each time you have assessed the geriatric patient, you note multiple bruises and dehydration. Upon reviewing his history with both residents, you always receive conflicting stories. What do you suspect?
    a. Probable senile dementia
    b. Possible elder abuse and neglect
    c. Probable TIA
    d. Probable leukemia

80. Which of the following is the medical term for a nosebleed?
    a. Epidermis
    b. Rhinoplasty
    c. Epistaxis
    d. Perfusion

81. What is the term that is used for hypoperfusion resulting from the massive loss of blood?
   a. Hypovolemic shock
   b. Hemorrhagic shock
   c. Cardiogenic shock
   d. Electrical shock

82. What is the volume of blood in a normal adult?
   a. 2 to 4 liters
   b. 1 to 3 liters
   c. 8 to 10 liters
   d. 5 to 7 liters

83. You arrive at a multiple-vehicle accident and prepare to transport an injured patient who states that he cannot feel his legs. Upon examination of his lower extremities, you notice that both legs appear to have dilated veins. What do you suspect?
   a. Anaphylactic shock
   b. Septic shock
   c. Hypovolemic shock
   d. Neurogenic shock

84. When you assess a patient's blood loss, which of the following is inaccurate?
   a. The smaller the patient, the less blood volume is present
   b. The smaller the patient, the lower the amount of bleeding that will cause shock
   c. A child loses blood at a slower rate than an adult does
   d. A young adult tolerates blood loss better than an adult does

85. How can you determine if a laceration involves an artery or a vein?
   a. A vein bleeds bright red blood with high pressure
   b. A vein bleeds dark red blood, steadily, but with low pressure
   c. An artery bleeds bright red blood, with low pressure
   d. A vein oozes slowly

86. You arrive at the scene of a car vs. pedestrian accident and observe that the victim has a major laceration of the thigh with extensive bleeding. He is lying on the ground and appears unresponsive. What is your first action?
   a. Don protective gloves, and apply direct pressure on the wound
   b. Don protective gloves, and assess the airway and breathing
   c. Don protective gloves, and start CPR
   d. Don protective gloves, and apply an upper thigh tourniquet

87. Your teenage patient has a nosebleed and appears extremely distraught. Which of the following treatment methods is inappropriate?
   a. Lean the patient forward
   b. Pinch the fleshy skin at the lower portion of the nose
   c. Place the patient in the Trendelenburg position (lying back with feet up)
   d. Keep the patient calm and quiet

88. You respond to a car accident involving a nine-year-old boy. During your assessment of the child, you observe that his abdomen is rigid and tender with slight bruising at the site where the seat belt restrained him. Based on these findings, what is your main concern?
    a. Fractured ribs
    b. Fractured sternum
    c. Internal bleeding
    d. Punctured lung

89. A call comes in for a child who was in a sledding accident and has a large abdominal laceration. Upon arrival at the scene, you open the girl's coat and see intestines protruding from her abdominal wound. What is the medical term for this?
    a. Penetration wound
    b. Crush injury
    c. Hematoma
    d. Evisceration

90. Which of the following is a closed injury?
    a. Hematoma
    b. Laceration
    c. Amputation
    d. Abrasion

91. What is the name for a closed injury in which there is cellular damage under the dermis with discoloration?
    a. Laceration
    b. Abrasion
    c. Concussion
    d. Contusion

92. You respond to an emergency call at a local factory in which a woman entangled her hair in a piece of machinery. As you approach the victim, you observe that a portion of her scalp with the hair attached has come off and is hanging from the equipment. Which of the following is the medical term for this type of injury?
    a. Avulsion
    b. Abrasion
    c. Laceration
    d. Amputation

93. When you assess a patient with a penetrating soft-tissue wound, what do you check for in addition to the original injury?
    a. Exit wound
    b. Fracture
    c. Burn
    d. Contusion

94. An injury to the lung that results in a sucking chest wound requires which of the following types of dressings?
a. Compression
b. Occlusive taped on four sides
c. Bulky
d. Occlusive taped on three sides

95. When a patient has an open abdominal wound with evisceration, what type of dressing do you apply?
a. Dry sterile gauze, covered with Vaseline gauze, then a compression dressing
b. Sterile gauze, moistened with sterile saline or water, covered with Vaseline gauze (occlusive)
c. Replace organs into the abdomen, then apply Vaseline gauze
d. Sterile bulky dressing to keep wound from further eviscerating

96. Sunburn is usually superficial and involves one layer of the epidermis. What is the classification of the common sunburn?
a. Second-degree burn
b. First-degree burn
c. Full-thickness burn
d. Third-degree burn

97. What is the main concern for a patient who has suffered burns to the head and neck?
a. Disfiguring scarring
b. Contractions
c. Airway involvement
d. Sinus burns

98. You arrive at the scene of an injury from a downed electrical wire. As you assess a victim, you find only small entrance and exit wounds. What is your first response?
a. Apply dressings and release the patient
b. Possible internal injuries—treat local wounds and transport
c. Do not touch the patient until she is free from the electrical source
d. Administer oxygen

99. When calculating the burn area of an adult, the head and neck are 9% of the body surface area, each upper extremity is 9%, the back and abdomen are each 18%, each leg is 18%, and the genitalia is 1%. What is the medical term for this formula?
a. "9-9-9"
b. "Critical burn rule"
c. "Eighteen percent rule"
d. "Rule of nines"

100. What is the name of the document that explains the type of chemical and first-aid care for that chemical exposure?
a. Chemical information sheet (CIS)
b. *Physicians' Desk Reference* (PDR)
c. Material safety data sheet (MSDS)
d. Poison control data (PCD)

101. You respond to an emergency call for an unresponsive child. At the scene, you notice an empty nail polish remover bottle on the floor. If a child ingests a chemical, which call do you make first?
   a. ER
   b. 911
   c. Poison control center
   d. The pediatrician

102. When do you classify a burn as critical?
   a. Full-thickness, covering 10% of the body, or partial-thickness, covering 30%
   b. Full-thickness, covering 7% of the body, or partial-thickness, covering 20%
   c. Full-thickness, covering 30% of the body, or partial-thickness, covering 20%
   d. Full-thickness, covering 5% of the body, or partial-thickness, covering 10%

103. Emergency care for the burn patient includes which of the following treatments:
   a. Apply cold sterile saline or sterile water to the burn
   b. Cover the burn with clean dry dressing
   c. Apply ointment to the burn to soothe and prevent scarring
   d. Keep the patient cool during transport to prevent additional burn damage

104. You arrive at the scene of a fall from a balcony. The teenage victim is writhing in pain from a broken leg. As you inspect the limb, you notice that the tibia and fibula are broken in many places. What is the name for this type of fracture?
   a. Greenstick
   b. Spiral
   c. Comminuted
   d. Stress

105. The average pulse for a five-year-old falls within what range?
   a. 70 to 115
   b. 60 to 80
   c. 120 to 160
   d. 160 to 170

106. In an infant or child, what organ is proportionally larger than that of an adult and may cause an airway obstruction?
   a. Larynx
   b. Tongue
   c. Uvula
   d. Cricoid ring

107. You arrive at the home of a six-year-old boy who is sitting up, leaning forward, and his nostrils are flared. What do these signs indicate?
   a. High fever
   b. Difficulty breathing
   c. Anxiety
   d. Panic attack

108. During the same visit to the child's home, you hear a loud harsh sound when the boy inhales. What is the name of this sound?
    a. Asthma
    b. Bronchitis
    c. Pneumonia
    d. Stridor

109. When you arrive at the home of a nine-year-old boy who has a peanut allergy, the mother informs you that the boy accidentally ingested a cookie from a facility that also uses peanuts in foods. The boy has hives and states that he has an itchy tongue. What is your next action?
    a. Administer his epinephrine autoinjector, apply oxygen, then transport
    b. Start oxygen and transport
    c. Apply topical corticosteroid cream, and instruct his mother to watch him
    d. Give ice water, apply corticosteroid cream, and then transport

110. You enter the home of the mother of an 18-month-old baby. She frantically recounts that she stepped out of the bathroom for a phone call. Upon her return, the baby was submerged and blue. What is your first action?
    a. Assess the baby for pulse and respirations; if applicable, begin CPR
    b. Report the mother for child endangerment
    c. Apply oxygen and transport the baby
    d. Wrap the baby in warm blankets and transport

111. During a professional baseball game, a ball hit a 10-year-old boy in the left lower back. When you assess the child, you notice bruising and swelling over the kidney area. What is your main concern?
    a. Subdural hematoma
    b. Internal bleeding
    c. Fractured spine
    d. Fractured ribs

112. You respond to a call for a child who pulled a pot of boiling soup off the stove. When you assess the three-year-old, you observe blistering over his entire face, neck, and trunk of the body. What is your main goal?
    a. Ensure a patent airway and transport immediately
    b. Apply sterile saline or water, sterile dressings, and then transport
    c. Apply antibiotic ointment, dry dressing, and then transport
    d. Wrap in warm blankets, transport

113. Why is the head tilt contraindicated in establishing a patent airway in an infant?
    A. The infant's head is small and easily moves out of position
    B. The infant's neck is weak and cannot hold the head in this position
    C. The infant's head is large, and this position can obstruct the airway
    D. The infant may roll to the side

114. If a child is afraid of having an oxygen mask placed directly on their face, what is an alternate method?
    a. Nasal airway
    b. Endotracheal tube
    c. Oral airway
    d. Blow-by oxygen

115. Which arteries do you use to assess the pulses of an infant?
    a. Brachial and temporal arteries
    b. Brachial and femoral arteries
    c. Carotid and femoral arteries
    d. Carotid and temporal arteries

116. Signs of respiratory arrest in an infant differ from those of an adult. Which of the following signs indicate respiratory arrest in an infant?
    a. Breathing rate less than 15 breaths per minute, slow heart rate
    b. Breathing rate less than 10 breaths per minute, limp muscle tone
    c. Breathing rate less than 20 breaths per minute, fast heart rate
    d. Breathing rate less than 30 breaths per minute, slow heart rate

117. What is the leading cause of death in children and adolescents?
    a. Drowning
    b. Poisoning
    c. Trauma
    d. Infection

118. You respond to a call for a nine-year-old with a possible fractured arm. As you approach the house, you realize that you have been on multiple calls to this address. Your assessment of the child reveals small burns and multiple bruises in various stages of healing, in addition to the deformity of the arm. The child is quiet and withdrawn. What is your response?
    a. Accuse the parents of child abuse and then transport the child for treatment
    b. Transport the child, and report your suspicions to your supervisor for notification of the proper agency
    c. Transport the child for treatment, and then call the police
    d. Write your report, including your opinion about the abuse

119. Which type of child abuse most frequently results in a lethal injury?
    a. Central nervous system injury, such as shaken baby syndrome
    b. Burns
    c. Fractures
    d. Puncture wounds

120. You arrive at the home of a young couple who have an unresponsive one-month-old baby. Upon examination, you see that the baby is in rigor mortis (the rigid stiffening of the muscles after death). What is your next action?
    a. CPR
    b. Intubate the baby, and then transport
    c. Comfort the parents
    d. Use the defibrillator, and then start CPR

Answers and Explanations

1. C: Body substance isolation precautions are necessary when suctioning a patient due to the likelihood of exposure to bodily fluids. When suctioning a patient's airway, the maximum time to apply the suction catheter is 15 seconds. Use a catheter that is appropriate for the situation, and do not insert it beyond the base of the tongue.

2. D: Measure the distance between the corner of the mouth and the earlobe.

3. A: The epiglottis is the flaplike structure that closes the entrance into the trachea (the glottis) and prevents food and liquids from entering the trachea. The uvula is a small V-shaped extension of the soft palate, which hangs in the center of the entrance to the throat, above the tongue. The cricoid ring is a complete cartilaginous circle of tissue located at the top of the trachea, just below the larynx. The diaphragm is a curved muscular membrane that separates the thoracic cavity from the abdominal cavity.

4. B: The rate of 12 to 20 breaths per minute is normal for an adult.

5. A: The patient's respiratory rate is within the normal range, but you observe that the chest wall is only moving slightly. This indicates inadequate tidal volume. The patient may have cyanosis, pneumonia, or bronchitis, but the description of the chest moving only slightly indicates an inadequate tidal volume. Additional information regarding symptoms and signs may indicate underlying conditions.

6. C: The most frequently seen symptom of respiratory distress is a change in the respiratory rate, either faster or slower. Cyanosis is a bluish cast of the skin and mucous membranes because of a low oxygen level. Absent respiratory sounds indicate respiratory failure. A change in consciousness may occur because of an inadequate level of oxygen to the brain, but it would not be the most commonly observed symptom of acute respiratory distress.

7. B: *Mouth-to-mask* is the ideal method for ventilating a nonbreathing patient. The bag-valve-mask (BVM) is a common technique seen in a hospital setting. It is most effective when used by a team of two EMTs. When there is only one EMT available to perform ventilation, the flow-restricted, oxygen-powered ventilation device is preferable in a nonbreathing adult. This technique is not suitable for an infant or child due to the possibility of lung tissue damage and air entering the stomach.

8. A: First, you should assume your position above the patient's head. If a second EMT is available to assist you, he or she should stabilize the head and neck. When working alone, use your knees to keep the head from moving. Use a mask, and preserve the seal by placing the thumb and index fingers on top of the mask, with the middle, ring, and little fingers placed firmly under the chin. Once the mask is in place, use the jaw thrust to open the airway. Do not apply pressure to the chin, because this may occlude the airway.

9. D: It is imperative to use a *water-soluble lubricant* when inserting any type of airway, because a petroleum-based lubricant could enter the lung and cause lipid pneumonia. The correct method for

measuring a nasopharyngeal airway is to measure the distance between the tip of the nose and the earlobe. Position the bevel of the airway toward the base of the nose or the septum.

10. B: If air is escaping through the nose and mouth, the immediate action is to close the mouth and pinch the nose.

11. C: When ventilating a trauma patient, use the jaw thrust to open the airway. A tracheotomy or an endotracheal tube may be necessary at some point, but the initial technique is the jaw thrust. The head tilt is not appropriate due to the possibility of cervical spine injury.

12. A: Oxygen tanks contain gas under very high pressure and may explode if ruptured. Always handle these tanks with care, and store in a manner that prevents movement when transporting. Wrapping the tanks with blankets is not a necessary precaution, but securing the tanks to prevent rolling or falling is essential. The valves and gauges are the most fragile parts of the tank, and they require extra care when transporting.

13. C: You form a general impression during the first few seconds of contact with the patient. The most important determination is the presence of any life-threatening condition or injury. If the patient is injured or ill, "sick" or "not sick," is initially determined by observing and you can prioritize and form a plan of action. At this point, you do not have adequate information to determine a diagnosis or transport the patient.

14. D: When the description of the patient includes "oriented times three," this is a reference to the patient's correct response to who he is, where he is, and what day it is. It does not refer to his inability to respond verbally or his recognition of family.

15. B: A nonobservable condition that a patient describes is a symptom. A sign is a medical or traumatic condition that someone other than the patient is able to observe and identify. Diagnosis refers to the identification of a disorder or illness through a physical examination, medical testing, or other procedures. A sensation is a physical feeling caused by having one or more of the sense organs stimulated.

16. C: A normal capillary refill time is less than two seconds.

17. B: When describing the area of an extremity that is near the trunk, the correct term is proximal. Distal refers to an area away, or distant, from the trunk. Posterior means toward the back, and lateral means away from the midline.

18. B: The prone position refers to lying on the abdomen. Lying on the back is the supine position. The Trendelenburg position and the shock position both involve lying back with the feet elevated; the shock position differs by having the patient bend at the hip. Lying back at a 45° angle is the Fowler's position.

19. C: Palpate carotid pulsations lateral to the larynx on both sides of the neck. The femoral arteries are located in the inguinal areas. There are no main arteries located in the axilla or posterior lateral neck.

20. D: The normal respiratory rate for an adult is 12 to 20 breaths per minute (BPM).

21. C: The posterior tibial and the dorsalis pedis arteries are preferable for use in assessing circulation in the lower extremities.

22. B: The nonrebreather mask is the preferred method for nonhospital delivery of high-concentration oxygen. This type of system is capable of delivering 90% oxygen when set at a 15 liter-per-minute flow rate. The nasal cannula is a low-flow device and is not as effective as an oxygen delivery system. An oxygen tent is an in-hospital type of oxygen delivery system in which a patient remains in an oxygen-filled environment while on bedrest. A ventilator is a system used to assist in breathing when a patient has a tracheostomy tube or endotracheal tube and is unable to breathe independently.

23. A: When a patient is cyanotic with or without the additional signs of cool and clammy skin, oxygen administration through a rebreather mask is required. The application of a warm blanket may be useful by increasing the temperature of the skin thereby decreasing the workload of the circulatory system, in case the patient is in shock. You would not perform CPR unless you ascertain that the patient has no pulse. You would not administer any liquid by mouth because you do not have a diagnosis at this time, and you could cause further injury to the patient.

24. C: Scene size up is the process of evaluating the surroundings to ensure your own safety prior to approaching the patient's location. Any situation in which exposure to bodily fluids is a possibility requires the use of body substance isolation precautions. Personal precautions such as eye protection, gown, shoe covers, masks, and gloves are included in body substance isolation precautions. Mechanism of injury refers to the determination of the cause of the trauma based on your evaluation of the scene plus information gained from family, friends, or bystanders.

25. A: If you suspect the apartment has carbon monoxide present, evacuate the patients, and then call for an additional unit to assist in treatment and transport.

26. B: The presence of arguing men indicates the possibility of personal injury to you. Wait for the police to secure the scene prior to proceeding to assess the injured man.

27. D: The acronym DCAP-BTLS is a memory aid for the eight components you evaluate when performing the rapid trauma assessment. The "P" refers to penetrations or punctures.

28. B: Deformity of an extremity is most frequently the result of a broken bone.

29. D: A scrape where the top layers of the skin are missing is an abrasion. A contusion is a bruise. A puncture is a wound that is deep and narrow. A laceration refers to a cut in the skin usually caused by a sharp object.

30. C: The medical term crepitation is the sound described as crackling or bones rubbing together. Croup is a common child's respiratory illness in which there is inflammation of the larynx and trachea and a narrowing of the airway just below the vocal chords, resulting in a "bark like" cough. Wheezing is a high-pitched whistling sound associated with labored breathing. Gurgling refers to the sound of liquid bubbling in the airway, and it requires immediate suctioning.

31. B: The location of the appendix is in the RLQ or right lower quadrant. The divisions of the abdomen include the RUQ, or right upper quadrant, the LUQ, or left upper quadrant, and the LLQ, or left lower quadrant.

32. A: Jugular veins, which are the large veins located on either side of the posterior neck, are usually invisible when a patient is in the sitting position. When the veins are visible while the patient is in the sitting position, this indicates increased circulatory pressure. In the supine position, the jugular veins normally distend. If these veins are flat when the patient is supine, it may signify blood loss.

33. C: The information you gain from your assessment and observation of the patient is the objective assessment. The subjective assessment refers to information attained from the patient, family members, or bystanders. The rapid assessment is a quick evaluation of the medical patient from head to toe, commonly requiring less than 90 seconds. Patient history is the term used for the acquired information about the patient.

34. D: The zygomatic arch is the formation that consists of a slender bar of bone found on each side of the face that connects the cheekbone to the temporal bone. Mandible is the medical term for the lower jawbone. Maxilla is the pair of bones that fuses at the midline to form the upper jawbone. The orbit is the round cavity in the skull in which the eye is located.

35. C: Assess and record vital signs of the stable patient every 15 minutes.

36. D: When you make an error on a report, strike through the mistake with a single horizontal line, initial beside the strikeout, and then write the correct information. Never erase, use correction fluid, or obliterate with multiple lines any information on a medical report.

37. B: The trade name is the name given to a medication by the manufacturer. The name listed in the United States Pharmacopeia for a medication is the generic name. Popular or pharmacology names are not proper medical terms.

38. A: Repeat the name, dosage, and route of administration to the physician to confirm his order.

39. B: Emphysema is a disease of the lungs in which the alveolar sacs enlarge and lose their flexibility and surface area. Asthma is a disease of the respiratory system with symptoms of coughing, wheezing, difficulty breathing, and a tight feeling in the chest. Stridor is a harsh high-pitched wheeze caused by obstruction of the air passages. Pneumonia is an inflammation of the lung caused by bacterium, a virus, or a chemical or physical irritant.

40. B: Oxygen is the first medication a patient in respiratory distress requires. If the patient has a physician-prescribed inhaler, you must obtain medical direction prior to assisting the patient in using it. Epinephrine (adrenaline) is a medication that is useful in the ER for a severe asthma attack. In a patient with congestive heart failure, the drug Lasix (furosemide) relieves lung congestion by reducing the fluid.

41. A: Angina is the medical term that describes chest pain that follows exertion and results from poor oxygenation of the cardiac muscle. Dyspnea refers to difficulty in breathing. Congestive heart failure is the term used for a form of heart failure in which the heart is unable to pump out the returning blood quickly enough, resulting in congestion in the veins and fluid build-up in the lungs. Tachycardia is the medical term for a fast heart rate.

42. C: The carotid arteries are located on either side of the neck, and they supply blood to the head and brain. The temporal arteries lie on either side of the head at the temple area. Jugular veins

return blood from the head and brain to the heart. Popliteal arteries lie on the posterior aspect of the knees.

43. D: Your immediate suspicion should be that this patient has the signs and symptoms of shock. After further assessment, the patient's injuries may include broken bones, head injuries, or heart attack, but the signs and symptoms initially point to shock.

44. B: The body attempts to compensate for shock by maintaining the blood pressure in a normal range for as long as possible. When a patient exhibits signs and symptoms of shock, even if her blood pressure reading is within a normal range, you treat the patient for shock. The patient may be hypothermic, but complete treatment for shock should be implemented, which may include a warming blanket and IV hydration therapy.

45. A: Nitroglycerin, available in sublingual tablets and spray, is the medication of choice for treating angina. Oxygen is a gas, and the usual routes of administration are by mask or nasal cannula. Digitalis is a medication used for regulating the heart rate. Lasix (furosemide) is a drug used for eliminating excess fluid from the body.

46. B: After administering nitroglycerin, instruct the patient to allow the medication to dissolve under her tongue, keeping her mouth closed. Check the B/P within two minutes. Do not have the patient rinse her mouth. Defibrillation is only used when ventricular fibrillation is present and not as a treatment for angina.

47. C: Defibrillation makes the greatest difference in survival of the cardiac arrest patient. IV therapy and oxygen administration are important, but the most important action is defibrillation. Nitroglycerin is a drug used for relief of angina.

48. D: Stabbing pain in the chest that increases in intensity with deep breaths is usually associated with the respiratory system. Cardiac pain is characteristically a crushing or pressure type of discomfort. GI upset and gallbladder disease may cause pain in the center of the chest or back or under the right rib cage.

49. B: These are signs and symptoms of cardiac compromise, which include a feeling of pressure or squeezing pain in the chest that may radiate to one or both arms, the neck, jaw, or upper back. Diaphoresis (sweating) and shortness of breath are common. The patient may express anxiety and fear of death or impending doom. The pulse and blood pressure are often abnormal, and the patient may experience nausea or vomiting. If the patient were experiencing a cardiac arrest, he would be unresponsive. A panic attack is a sudden overpowering feeling of fear that may prevent the patient from functioning as normal. When a patient has a bleeding ulcer, he may have bloody emesis, tarry black stools, and low blood pressure.

50. B: If any pulse is palpable, do not use the AED. It is appropriate to use when the patient is unresponsive and there is no detectable pulse or respiration.

51. D: Fibrillation is the condition in which the heart muscle fibers are producing uncontrolled rapid contractions. During fibrillation, the heart cannot produce a pulse. Ventricular tachycardia refers to a heart rate of more than 100 beats per minute in which the beat originates in the ventricles. Atrial tachycardia is a condition in which the beat originates in the atrium and the rate per minute is above the normal range. Heart block is a condition in which the nerve impulses that

control the heartbeat are irregular, and this causes the atria and ventricles to stop beating in the same rhythm.

52. B: A low white blood count could prevent the patient from having the ability to fight infections. Anemia is the condition in which there is an inadequate amount of red blood cells or the existing red cells are deficient in hemoglobin. Uncontrolled bleeding may result from a low platelet count. Blood clotting may be the result of an injury to a blood vessel or slow circulation that results in clot formation.

53. C: Red blood cells contain hemoglobin that carries oxygen to the tissues of the body. Hemoglobin is an iron-containing protein found in red blood cells that enables the transport of oxygen to the tissues. Plasma is the fluid component of the blood that transports the various types of cells.

54. A: Altered mental status is the condition in which a patient responds inappropriately, either verbally or nonverbally. A seizure is a sudden attack caused by a random discharge of electrical current in the brain; it usually results in a temporary altered mental status. A coma is a prolonged episode of deep unconsciousness. Hypoglycemia is a serious and sudden drop in blood sugar levels in which the patient may appear to be intoxicated, shaky, diaphoretic, and clammy.

55. B: There are several possible causes of seizures, including fever, infection, intoxication, poisoning, hypoglycemia, head trauma, hypoxia, and epilepsy. Encourage all seizure patients to go to the emergency room for additional examination by a physician.

56. A: This patient has the signs of hyperglycemia (high blood glucose) and diabetic coma. This patient may be an insulin-dependent diabetic, and because refrigeration is necessary for insulin, it is logical to search the refrigerator for this drug. Orange juice and administration of IV glucose are appropriate for hypoglycemia (low blood glucose) to increase the blood glucose level. This patient is not responsive, but she does have a pulse and is breathing, so CPR is not appropriate.

57. C: A blood glucose level of 80 mg/dL or lower indicates hypoglycemia, or low blood glucose. A normal reading for blood glucose level is 80 to 120 mg/dL. Hyperglycemia is an extremely high glucose level. Diabetes is the general term for the medical condition that prevents insulin production or effective metabolism.

58. B: Never administer oral glucose to an unconscious patient who cannot protect their airway.

59. C: The preeminent sign of hypoperfusion is the change in mental status.

60. A: Anaphylaxis is the term used for a severe allergic reaction.

61. B: The boy is loudly wheezing and has facial edema; both of these signs indicate a severe allergic reaction. Because the boy's physician ordered the epinephrine autoinjector pen, call for medical direction and then administer the medication. The child is already having signs of respiratory distress, and without intervention he may progress into full anaphylactic shock. The child may know how to give himself the injection, but because he is already having difficulty breathing, the better choice would be to get medical direction, then administer the drug.

62. B: Oxygen is the first treatment for a patient who had inhaled toxin exposure.

63. D: Do not attempt to collect a venomous snake or spider for identification.

64. A: Activated charcoal acts by binding to certain poisons and keeping them from being absorbed in the stomach.

65. C: When treating a patient with hypothermia, remove the patient from the cold, disrobe of any wet clothing, and cover with a blanket, handle the patient gently, administer high-flow warmed and humidified oxygen, do not give stimulating foods or drinks, do not massage the extremities, use warm IV fluids, and check the pulse for at least 30 to 45 seconds before initiating CPR.

66. C: A patient in the late stages of hypothermia will present with pale, cyanotic skin.

67. D: Deep-tissue damage from exposure to cold presents with signs and symptoms of white, waxy skin; firm or frozen feel upon palpation; possible swelling or blisters; lack of feeling; and, if it is thawed, the skin appears flushed, red or purple, mottled, pale, or cyanotic.

68. C: When a hyperthermic patient has skin that feels hot and has an altered mental status, apply cool packs to the neck, axilla, and groin; fan the patient in an air-conditioned ambulance; keep the patient's skin *wet* by applying water with sponges or wet towels; and transport to the hospital immediately.

69. C: Remove the patient from the water after placing him on a long backboard and securing his head with a cervical spine immobilization device or with manual stabilization of the head.

70. A: The stage of labor in which the head of the baby is showing in the vaginal orifice is crowning. Pushing is the term used for the act of bearing down as if having a bowel movement. Bloody show refers to the expulsion of the mucous plug because of cervical dilation in the beginning of labor. Dilation is the act of opening of the cervix during labor to allow for expulsion of the baby.

71. B: The medical term for the unborn developing baby is fetus. A zygote is the fertilized female egg. Newborn is the name given to the infant from birth up to a few weeks of age. Infant is a very young child that can neither walk nor talk.

72. A: Once pulsations in the cord have stopped, clamp the cord around four finger widths from the baby's body, then again four to five inches from the first clamp.

73. B: When the infant's head delivers, immediately check to see if the umbilical cord is around its neck. If the cord is around the neck, try to loosen and slide it over the head. If it is too tight to remove, clamp it in two places, and carefully cut between the clamps. You cannot deliver a baby with the cord around its neck. Doing nothing is not appropriate: clamp the cord in two places and cut it. Never cut the cord without first clamping it.

74. C: Never pull on the umbilical cord. The placenta delivers on its own, usually within 30 minutes of delivery. Encourage the mother to push with contractions.

75. B: A birth in which the buttocks or legs deliver first is a breech presentation. Cephalic presentation refers to the delivery of the head first. Prolapsed cord is the situation in which the umbilical cord presents before the rest of the baby's body. Premature birth is the name given to a baby born less than 37 weeks after conception or weighing less than 5.5 pounds.

76. C: Almost half of the elderly patients suffering from an acute myocardial infarction (MI) present in the ER with shortness of breath as their only symptom. Chest pain, nausea, numbness in the arm, sweating, abdominal pain, and fatigue are all symptoms of MI and may be present.

77. C: Dementia is the medical term for the neurological disorder that results in the loss of higher functions of the brain. Syncope is another term for fainting. Vertigo means dizziness in which the patient may complain of a loss of balance, a whirling sensation, loss of balance, or lightheadedness. A TIA, or transient ischemic attack, is the term used for a temporary interruption in blood flow to a portion of the brain. The TIA, or mini-stroke, may be the precursor for a major stroke.

78. D: "Coffee-ground" emesis is the classic sign of bleeding from the stomach. Bleeding from the colon may be red or black and tarry in appearance. Hematuria is the term for bleeding from the bladder, which causes the urine to appear pink. Hemoptysis refers to bloodstained sputum from the respiratory system.

79. B: When you have multiple incidences of unexplained bruising and dehydration and conflicting stories of how these injuries occurred, you consider elder abuse and neglect as a possible cause. Senile dementia may be present, but none of these symptoms point to this condition. A transient ischemic attack (TIA) presents with the symptoms of stroke. Leukemia patients often have bruising, but the combination of history and physical findings indicate a possibility of abuse.

80. C: Epistaxis is the medical term for nosebleed. Epidermis refers to the outer layer of the skin. Rhinoplasty is the term use for plastic surgery of the nose. Perfusion is circulation of the blood to all the tissues of the body, delivering oxygen and nutrients and removing wastes.

81. B: Hemorrhagic shock is the medical term for hypoperfusion due to a massive hemorrhage (loss of blood). Hypovolemic shock differs from hemorrhagic shock in that the volume in the circulatory system is low due to the loss of bodily fluid from dehydration, diarrhea, vomiting, or significant burns. Cardiogenic shock refers to hypoperfusion due to a cardiac cause.

82. D: The normal adult has a total blood volume of five to seven liters.

83. D: When a patient has a spinal cord injury, the blood vessels below the injury site stop constricting and dilate due to neurogenic shock. Anaphylactic shock is the result of a severe allergic reaction. Septic shock occurs in the presence of an overwhelming infection. Hypovolemic shock is hypoperfusion due to fluid volume loss from diarrhea, dehydration, vomiting, or significant burns.

84. C: A child loses blood at the same rate as an adult, so the same wound can be much more serious in a child.

85. B: A lacerated vein steadily bleeds dark red blood. An artery bleeds rapidly, and the blood is bright red.

86. B: After donning protective gloves, assure that the patient has an open airway and ventilation, and then address the laceration by applying concentrated direct pressure. Apply a tourniquet only if directed to do so by a physician. If the patient is in cardiac arrest, then CPR is appropriate.

87. C: The initial treatment for epistaxis is the application of pressure (pinching) to the nostrils, because most nosebleeds originate in the anterior portion of the nose. Lean the patient forward to

prevent blood from going down the throat. Do not have the patient lie back in the Trendelenburg position; the increased blood pressure to the head would exacerbate the bleeding. Keep the patient calm and quiet to decrease the blood pressure. If the nosebleed does not stop with applied pressure, the patient may need nasal packing in the ER.

88. C: Based on the abdominal rigidity and tenderness in addition to the slight bruising from the seatbelt restraint, internal bleeding may be present. Fractured ribs, sternum, and punctured lungs would have a different set of signs and symptoms.

89. D: Evisceration is the medical term for the protrusion of any organs from a wound. The word viscera refers to internal organs. Penetration or puncture wound denotes an injury in which an object pushed through the skin into the soft tissue. A crush wound or crush injury is one that is the result of blunt force trauma.

90. A: A hematoma is a closed injury in which a large amount of blood collects under the skin. Laceration, amputation, and abrasion are all open injuries.

91. D: A contusion, or bruise, is a closed injury of the soft tissue in which there is cellular damage and discoloration of the dermis. Laceration and abrasion are both open injuries. Concussion is a closed injury involving the brain.

92. A: Avulsion is the term used to describe an open wound in which tissue completely tears away from the body. Abrasion is an open wound that results from a scrape of the dermis. Laceration is another name for a cut. Amputation is the separation of an appendage from the rest of the body.

93. A: When you encounter a soft-tissue wound, especially a penetrating injury, always examine the opposite side of the patient for an exit wound. You observe for burns, fractures, and contusions as part of your normal assessment, not as a response to a penetrating soft-tissue injury.

94. D: A sucking chest wound requires an occlusive dressing taped on three sides to limit air from entering the lung, but it allows air to escape. Compression dressings prevent additional bleeding. Bulky dressings not only aid in reducing blood loss, but they also provide stabilization.

95. B: The proper dressing for a wound with evisceration of internal organs is sterile gauze, moistened with sterile water or saline to keep the viscera from becoming dry. Place an occlusive dressing, such as Vaseline gauze, over the sterile moistened gauze, to maintain the moisture content. Never attempt to replace the organs into the abdomen. Position the patient with the knees flexed, if not contraindicated by a spinal injury, to prevent stretching of the abdominal muscles and further evisceration. Dry dressings would adhere to the viscera. Bulky dressings would apply pressure and possibly force the viscera back into the abdominal cavity, increasing the risk of infection.

96. B: Sunburn is usually superficial, involving only the epidermis and is a first-degree burn. A second-degree or partial thickness burn involves both the dermis and epidermis. A full-thickness or third-degree burn involves all layers of the epidermis, dermis, and subcutaneous layer and possibly muscle, bone, and nerves.

97. C: The major concern for a patient with burns on the face and neck is the airway. When the patient has burns in these areas, there is the possibility that the patient inhaled smoke and may deteriorate due to throat swelling and impaired breathing.

98. C: Prior to touching the patient, make sure that the electrical source is absent, so you are not at risk for shock. Once the scene is safe, treat the patient, keeping in mind that the entrance and exit wounds may appear minimal, but internal damage is a possibility.

99. D: The "rule of nines" assigns a value of 9% to each arm and the head and neck, 18% to the abdomen and to the back, 18% to each leg, and 1% to the genitalia.

100. C: All industrial facilities must keep material safety data sheets (MSDSs) that describe the chemicals they use and the first-aid treatments for exposure to those chemicals.

101. C: The first call you should make is to the poison control center, follow their instructions, and then transport the patient with the poison container to the ER.

102 A: A critical burn is one in which there is a full-thickness burn of 10% or more of the body surface area or a partial-thickness burn of 30% or more of the body surface area.

103. B: Use room-temperature sterile water or saline to stop the burning process. Cover the burn with a clean, dry dressing. Do not apply ointments, lotions, or antiseptics, and avoid opening any blisters. Keep the patient warm during transport.

104. C: A fracture in which there are multiple breaks is a comminuted fracture. A greenstick fracture is bone damage in a child where the bone is bent. A spiral fracture is the result of a twisting injury. A stress fracture is the consequence of multiple injuries to the same bone, as in a running injury.

105. A: The correct range for the pulse of a five-year-old is 70 to 115.

106. B: The tongue is proportionally larger in the infant and child and may occlude the airway more easily than the tongue of an adult.

107. B: These are signs of difficulty breathing.

108. D: A harsh loud sound heard during breathing is stridor. This patient may suffer from bronchitis, asthma, or pneumonia, but the type of sound he is making is called stridor.

109. A: The child is experiencing an allergic reaction, which can be life threatening. Administer the epinephrine autoinjector, apply oxygen, and transport the patient to the ER for further treatment and observation.

110. A: Because the baby is cyanotic, it is probable that it has no respirations or pulse. Assess the vital signs and if applicable, start CPR. The mother may be guilty of child neglect; the ER physicians may choose to report her to authorities, but at this point, the child is in a life-threatening situation and needs immediate intervention. Administer CPR first to attempt to revive the child. All other treatments, such as warm blankets, are secondary to reestablishing a pulse and respirations.

111. B: The ball hit the boy in the left lower back, and the bruising could indicate internal bleeding. Subdural hematoma is an injury to the head in which there is bleeding under the dura. There is no indication of fractures of the ribs, which is very painful, or injury to the spine, because the impact was to the left of the center of the back.

112. A: This child has a critical burn, so you establish an airway and transport him immediately. You can perform all other treatments en route.

113. C: The infant's head is large in comparison with its body, and the head tilt position could actually obstruct the airway. Position the head only far enough back so the bottom of the nose points straight up. The neck is weak, and the infant may roll, but the reason for avoiding the full head tilt is the potential obstruction of the airway.

114. D: The blow-by oxygen technique is an alternative for administering oxygen to a child who is afraid of having a mask on their face. Nasal and oral airways or endotracheal tubes are applicable only if the child is unresponsive.

115. B: Assess the pulse of an infant by palpating the brachial or femoral arteries.

116. B: Signs of respiratory arrest in an infant include a breathing rate of less than 10 breaths per minute, limp muscle tone, unresponsive, slow or absent heart rate, and weak or absent pulse.

117. C: The main cause of death in children and adolescents is trauma.

118. B: Your main objective is the treatment of the child. Report the suspected abuse to your supervisor. Record the injuries and factual information regarding the child's environment and any comments made by the parents or caregivers in quotes, keep a copy for yourself, and give a copy to your supervisor to present to the proper authorities.

119. A: Central nervous system injuries, such as shaken baby syndrome, are the most lethal types of child abuse injuries.

120. C: If the baby is in rigor mortis, do not attempt resuscitation. Observe the scene details, and document it carefully. Comfort the parents, and then contact your medical base to determine transfer protocol.